ANAESTHETICS, RESUSCITATION AND INTENSIVE CARE

A Textbook for Students and Residents

ANAESTHETICS RESUSCITATION AND INTENSIVE CARE

A Textbook for Students and Residents

WALTER NORRIS
M.D., F.F.A.R.C.S.

DONALD CAMPBELL
M.B., Ch.B., F.F.A.R.C.S., D.A.
Consultant Anaesthetists, Glasgow Royal Infirmary
Clinical Teachers in Anaesthetics
University of Glasgow

FOREWORD BY

JOHN W. DUNDEE
M.D., Ph.D., F.F.A.R.C.S., F.F.A.R.C.S.I.
Professor of Anaesthetics, The Queen's University of Belfast

THIRD EDITION

REPRINT

CHURCHILL LIVINGSTONE
EDINBURGH AND LONDON
1972

ISBN 0 443 00750 0

First Edition 1965

Second Edition 1968

Third Edition 1971

Reprinted 1972

Printed in Great Britain

FOREWORD

In recommending a book for use by medical students and housemen one should perhaps justify their learning something about anaesthesia and its ever widening field of non-theatre activities.

In many parts of the English-speaking world, general anaesthesia is now in the hands of specialist or trainee-specialist anaesthetists. While the advantages of this cannot be overemphasised from both the surgeon's and patient's point of view, it is unfortunate that, in Great Britain at least, the newly qualified doctor gets little opportunity of handling and caring for the anaesthetised patient. Most undergraduates simply fulfil the requirements of their particular medical school with regard to the administration of anaesthetics and are naturally unwilling to devote more than the minimum time to the subject in an already overcrowded curriculum. Thus they miss an opportunity of gaining first-hand experience of dealing with patients who have been made comatose and who may have induced respiratory or circulatory depression. There is no place where these states, which require the urgent attention of every doctor, can be seen so frequently and where their treatment is so successful as during anaesthesia or the immediate post-operative period.

No book can fill the place of practical experience in the operating room, recovery ward, intensive care, and respiratory units, but Drs Norris and Campbell have prepared the present volume so that the limited time which can be allocated to anaesthesia and allied topics will be spent to the best advantage. It contains a clear concise account of the different types of anaesthesia and the simplest and most reliable means by which these can be produced. Such a text could so easily develop into a "do it yourself" recipe book, but the authors have avoided this temptation by including adequate data on the pertinent physiology and pharmacology.

On such a sound foundation, the writers have based a valuable section on modern methods of resuscitation. This alone could recommend the book not only to students and house staff but to all physicians who are becoming increasingly aware of the immediate treatment of cardiovascular collapse. While avoiding controversial topics, this section deals fully with such important aspects as pH control and is presented with such clarity and simplicity as to be helpful to readers of all types.

The anaesthetist should be in a particularly favourable position with regards to knowledge on relief of post-operative pain. Drs Norris and Campbell have included precise instructions on the management of this important topic which will save many embarrassing moments for the " houseman " and be of inestimable value to the patient. Although it would take a book many times the size of the present one to deal adequately with all aspects of analgesia and pain relief, the basic knowledge in the present volume is a good foundation on which interested doctors could build such information. As the anaesthetist's interest in the patient should start with his pre-operative preparation and ordering of pre-anaesthetic medication, so this book covers all topics from the drugs given before operation to the long-term management of respiratory insufficiency.

It is not surprising that since the majority of anaesthetic text books cater for the potential specialist they contain too much detail for other readers. In addition they usually present both sides of controversial arguments, necessitating some experience in understanding the various views expressed and their relevance to the circumstances under which the reader may be working. This defect is avoided in the present volume which is a valuable book not only for senior medical students and house surgeons or house physicians but a useful manual for the beginner in the first few months of his anaesthetic training.

JOHN W. DUNDEE.

Belfast, 1965.

PREFACE TO THE THIRD EDITION

Since publication of the second edition of this book we have had the benefit of further advice and criticism from colleagues in many parts of the world. In the light of this advice some sections have been expanded, some modified and others retained although they may appear outdated in countries where anaesthesia is highly developed.

Changes in equipment, methods and attitudes are reflected throughout the book.

We have resisted the temptation to expand individual sections of the book which might enhance its value for some readers in the hope that by so doing the book will continue to serve the overall purpose for which it was originally intended.

We are again indebted to our publishers, E. & S. Livingstone, for help and guidance in the preparation of this edition.

WALTER NORRIS.
DONALD CAMPBELL.

Glasgow, 1971.

PREFACE TO THE FIRST EDITION

The administration of anaesthetics in this country is now firmly established in the hands of the specialist anaesthetist. Indeed after qualification a doctor may never require to give an anaesthetic again if he does not wish to do so. Most doctors, however, in their hospital life and indeed outwith hospital, will at some time work in co-operation with members of the anaesthetic department staff. Surgeons, obstetricians and dentists, of course, are in daily contact with anaesthetists, physicians are meeting and working with them in the treatment of various chest diseases, and many other specialists also co-operate with them.

To the student we hope to offer a background to his practical teaching in the operating theatre and explain the " whys " of anaesthesia rather than to attempt to explain how to give an anaesthetic. If he wishes to learn how to give an anaesthetic, he must do this in the operating theatre and over the course of many weeks or even months. We hope also to show that the interests and work of the anaesthetist are not limited to the operating theatre.

To the resident in hospital we hope to explain how he may help the anaesthetist and thus his patients by careful pre-operative care of the patient and by thinking of the therapy he is using and the effect it may have on the anaesthetic later. We hope also he will realise that there are many ways in which the anaesthetist can help him and that there are times when he should call a consultant anaesthetist rather than a consultant surgeon or physician.

In many hospitals the resident will find himself dealing with patients in intensive care units, particularly those dealing with respiratory emergencies, both medical and surgical. This is a field of work where it is essential that everyone should know what is expected of him and what can be done to help severely disabled patients. It is essential that " the man on the spot " should be fully conversant with all the methods which are used.

No matter what path the student intends to follow, we feel that a thorough knowledge of methods of resuscitation will prove invaluable to him whether he practises in hospital, in general practice or in any other branch of medicine. Acute respiratory and cardiac failure may occur anywhere and the chance of survival of the patient depends entirely on the ability of those present to maintain or restart an efficient circulation and ventilation within a few minutes.

It is for this reason that we have dealt with resuscitation, intensive care, tracheal intubation and intravenous therapy in greater practical detail. As with the administration of anaesthetics, however, there is no substitute for practical training and experience.

Finally, we feel that a knowledge of the accidents and medico-legal hazards which are associated with anaesthesia, resuscitation and intensive care will impress on both students and residents the need for care in applying these techniques.

W. Norris.
D. Campbell

Glasgow, 1965.

ACKNOWLEDGEMENTS

WE are grateful to Professor John W. Dundee who has so kindly written the foreword to this book and given us valuable criticism and advice during its preparation.

To Professor Alex. C. Forrester we are indebted for the chapter he has contributed and for his encouragement.

Dr. John Gillies and Professor J. D. Robertson read the manuscript in the early stages of its preparation and we are grateful to them for their constructive criticism and advice.

For permission to reproduce illustrations we are grateful to:—

Messrs. E. & S. Livingstone: Figs. 10, 13, 24, 25, 26, 49, 96, 115, 116, 117, 118, 119 and some forty illustrations from *A Nurse's Guide to Anaesthetics, Resuscitation and Intensive Care* (4th edition 1969).

Messrs. John Sherratt & Son, publishers of the *British Journal of Anaesthesia* and Drs. G. M. Paterson, G. H. Hulands and Professor John Nunn: Fig. 17.

The Editor of *The British Medical Bulletin* and Dr. H. G. Epstein: Fig. 18.

The Editor of the *Proceedings of the Royal Society of Medicine* and Professor W. A. Mackey: Fig. 109A, B and C.

We also gratefully acknowledge the following who supplied us with illustrations or material for their production:—

Mr. Adrian Litton: Figs. 9A and B.

The British Oxygen Company Limited: Figs. 12, 14, 28A and B, 55, 56, 61, 62, 110, 113.

Dr. Ralph Thomson: Fig. 27.

The late Dr. James Eaton: Fig. 36.

Armour Pharmaceutical Company: Figs. 37, 40 and 41.

Brunswick Corporation (U.K.) Ltd.: Fig. 38.

Smith and Nephew—Southalls Ltd.: Fig. 39.

Pharmax Ltd.: Fig. 46.

Professor Alex. C. Forrester: Figs. 48, 80 and the illustrations in his chapter.

Portland Plastics Ltd.: Figs. 59 and 89.

Messrs. Medical and Industrial Equipment Ltd.: Figs. 68 and 111.
Mr. Gabriel Donald: Figs. 92 and 129.
Dr. A. B. M. Telfer: Figs. 96 and 129.
Abbott Laboratories: Fig. 112.
Messrs. Airmed Ltd.: Fig. 114.
Dr. Nimmo McKellar: Fig. 126.
Macarthys Ltd.: Fig. 135.

The Warning Notice in the Appendix is reproduced by permission of the Scottish Home and Health Department.

We are again indebted to Mr. Robin Callander for the time, patience and skill he has devoted to producing the diagrams and line drawings. The photographs are the work of the late Mr. Kelly, Mr. Burns and the staff of the Department of Medical Illustration, Glasgow Royal Infirmary, to whom we are also indebted for their time, patience and skill.

Finally we are grateful to Dr. W. L. M. Baird and Miss E. H. Polley who have painstakingly read the proofs of this third edition.

LIST OF CONTENTS

CHAPTER I

ANALGESIA AND ANAESTHESIA

METHODS AND MODES OF ACTION

It is perhaps best to start by defining two commonly used terms, " analgesia " and " anaesthesia ".

Analgesia means absence of pain.

Anaesthesia means absence of all sensation.

The term analgesia is therefore correctly used to describe the state where pain has been abolished but other sensations remain and the patient is still conscious. Anaesthesia, on the other hand, is usually restricted to the state where all sensation is lost and the patient is unconscious.

The conduction of the painful impulses to the brain from a site of injury may be interrupted at any point between their origin and the sensory cortex (Fig. 1). It may also be interrupted in a variety of different ways. We are concerned with the use of drugs which do this, but these impulses may also be interrupted surgically by cutting the nerve supply to an area invaded by incurable painful tumour or, by dividing a tract in the spinal cord one may alleviate the pain caused by such a tumour. Tumours themselves may interrupt the passage of impulses along nerves and of course injury to the nerve such as follows some fractures, for example, has a similar effect. Extreme cold also blocks nerve conduction.

Drugs may be used to dull pain in two ways.

1. They may be deposited close to the nerves carrying the impulses to the brain. Thus drugs may be injected at the site of injury or in the line of the nerves as they pass through the tissues or even into the epidural or subarachnoid spaces to reach the area crossed by the nerves as they enter the cord. This type of drug, when brought into contact with a nerve, permeates into the nerve and stops conduction of the impulses at that point. This is therefore a local action.

2. Alternatively instead of attempting to block the passage of the painful impulse to the brain, it is possible to depress the brain which receives the impulse so that the pain is either felt

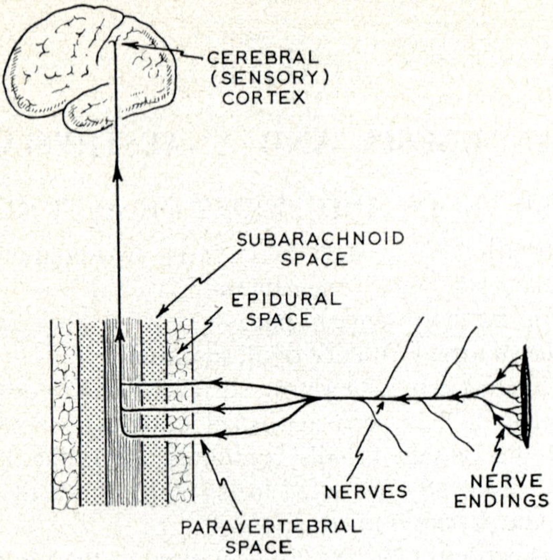

FIG. 1

The Pathway of Pain: The course of painful impulses from a wound to the brain is illustrated. The passage of the impulse can be interrupted at any of the sites indicated by the arrows.

with diminished intensity or not felt at all. The drugs which act in this way are of course not brought directly into contact with the brain by injection in that area, but are carried there in the blood stream. They may be administered by way of the stomach, the bowel, or the lungs (being absorbed into the blood stream) or they may be injected directly into a vein.

LOCAL OR REGIONAL ANALGESIA

Topical Application (Fig. 2)

Local analgesic solutions may be painted or sprayed on to mucous membranes or on to wound surfaces. In this way they are absorbed locally and produce analgesia of the area to which they have been applied. It must be emphasised that this method is ineffective where the solution is applied to unbroken skin as the drug is not absorbed and does not reach the nerve endings.

USES. This technique is mainly used in producing analgesia of the urethra, nose, throat and bronchial tree for examinations or minor surgical procedures. It is also of value in preparing a wound for subsequent cleansing and local infiltration. When a dilute solution of the analgesic drug is applied to the raw surface on a swab, this enables the wound to be cleaned and the discomfort of any subsequent local infiltration is minimised.

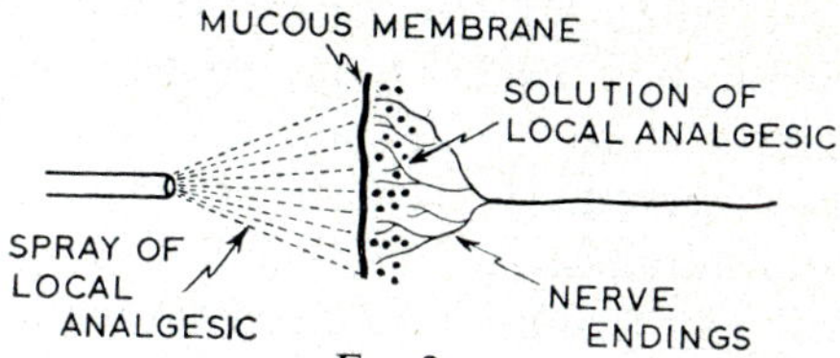

FIG. 2

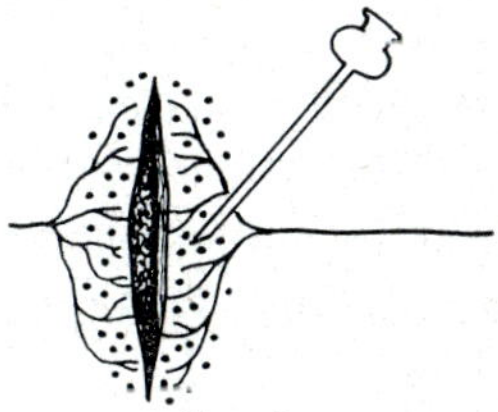

FIG. 3

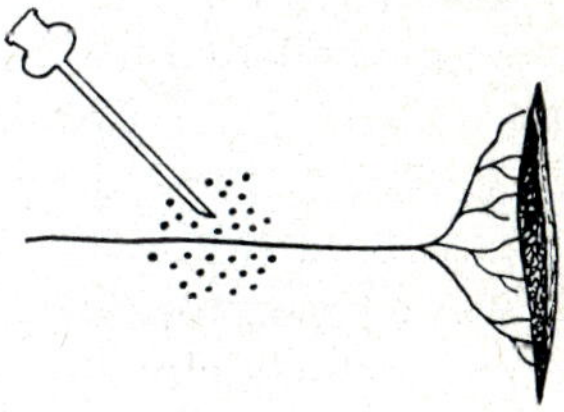

FIG. 4

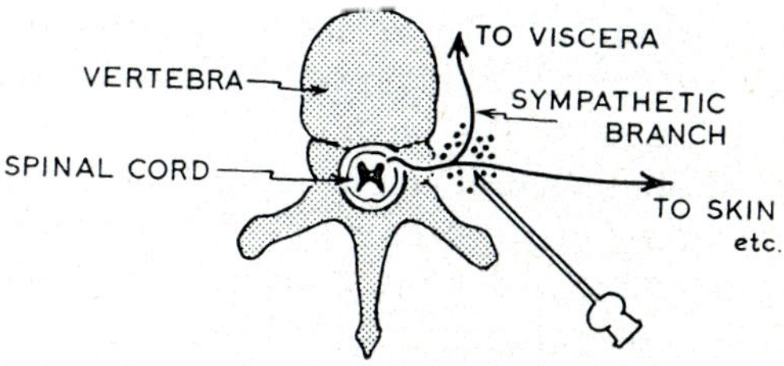

FIG. 5

FIGS. 2-5

Routes of administration of analgesics: Fig. 2. Topical application. Fig. 3. Local infiltration. Fig. 4. Regional nerve block. Fig. 5. Paravertebral nerve block.

Local Infiltration (Fig. 3)

Injection of a dilute analgesic solution in the area of the proposed operation will block the perception of pain at the level of the nerve endings. This is perhaps the simplest method of analgesia and is widely used for minor surgical operations.

If restricted to this type of case it is a safe procedure and has few if any after-effects so that the patient is able to eat and drink and return home shortly after operation. The method can be used for more extensive operations but then larger doses of the drug are necessary and thus side-effects are more likely. The safety margin is reduced. Extensive infiltration is also an unpleasant procedure for the patient. It is a common fallacy that local infiltration using dilute analgesic solutions is an entirely safe procedure. This is only true when two safeguards are carefully observed. In the first place great care must be taken to avoid administering an overdose. It is easy to forget that in extensive procedures considerable quantities of the drug may have been injected, albeit in dilute solution. Local analgesic agents have toxic properties as have other drugs and an overdose may be lethal (p. 224).

In the second place care must be taken to avoid intravascular injection of these drugs. Before and at intervals during the infiltration of the area of operation, aspiration through the syringe must be performed regularly to ensure that the needle does not lie within a blood vessel.

USES. This technique is commonly used for minor surgical procedures and is an excellent method for the surgeon working without the assistance of an anaesthetist. Provided the safeguards described are carefully observed, the technique is almost without complications. The method should not be used in the presence of local infection and is sometimes better avoided where the anatomy of the area may be distorted by the injection. This latter objection may be overcome by incorporating hyaluronidase in the solution.

Nerve Block (Fig. 4)

The main nerve which supplies the area of an operation can be blocked by injecting local analgesic solution close to it. Thus it is possible with a few injections to produce analgesia over a wide area. This is achieved by using quite small doses of the drug and may be less harmful than widespread infiltration. The technique has the advantage that the solution may be injected some distance proximal to the site of operation so that distortion of the anatomy is avoided and the presence of sepsis at the operative site is not a contra-indication.

USES. The technique is of particular value where the nerves which supply an area are easily accessible and by one or two injections, analgesia over quite a wide area may be achieved. It is of less value where the nerves are difficult of access.

The techniques described so far can be used for surgery on the extremities, head and neck and on the surface of the abdomen or thorax. If, however, it is intended to operate within the abdomen, the sympathetic branches which make up the nerve supply to the viscera must also be blocked.

Paravertebral Nerve Block (Fig. 5)

In this method the nerves are blocked close to the vertebrae before the sympathetic branch has left the main nerve. This technique can be used for surgical procedures inside the abdomen but as it involves multiple injections it is no longer popular for this type of case. Its use is therefore nowadays restricted to the blocking of a few nerves, such as the innervation of a leg, to produce vasodilatation in vascular disease.

The techniques described involve multiple injections and may cause the patient considerable discomfort where an extensive operation has to be performed. We will now therefore consider two techniques which by one single injection may produce analgesia over a wide area of the body.

Spinal or Subarachnoid Analgesia (Figs. 6 and 7)

Local analgesic solution introduced into the cerebrospinal fluid may be distributed widely to affect a large number of nerves. In this way by one injection, analgesia, muscular relaxation and sympathetic blockade affecting a large part of the body may be relatively easily produced.

The technique has many advantages.

1. Excellent analgesia results.
2. Muscular relaxation is also complete.
3. Sympathetic blockade is present. This produces not only a fall in blood pressure which may be advantageous in reducing haemorrhage at the operative site but also a contracted bowel which allows easy access to all parts of the abdomen.
4. The amount of solution which will produce a given area of analgesia can be readily estimated.

5. It is possible, though highly undesirable, for one person to perform the subarachnoid block and then perform the operation. This practice was a considerable advantage to surgeons when anaesthetists were unavailable.

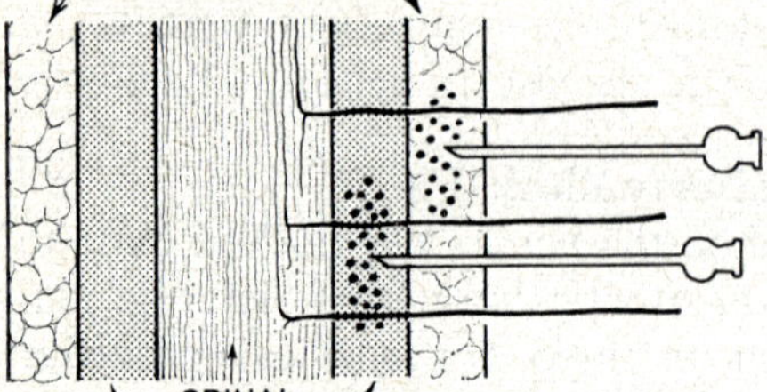

FIG. 6

Epidural and Spinal Analgesia: The diagram illustrates the two sites at which the analgesic solution is deposited, following introduction of the needle through the intervertebral space.

In view of these advantages it is at first sight surprising that the technique is not now commonly used, but most patients prefer to be asleep during operation and nowadays with trained anaesthetists widely available and the introduction of muscle relaxant drugs, a safe general anaesthetic can provide most of the advantages of spinal analgesia.

In the past spinal analgesia has been associated with a number of complications; some, which are minor in character, such as transient nerve palsy and headache, are relatively common while others, though less common, are severe, for example, paraplegia. Such complications have followed spinal analgesia given by competent anaesthetists using what have been apparently impeccable techniques. While headache is a minor complication in that it is never responsible for the patient's death, it may be severe and intractable and last for several days, making the patient extremely miserable. The occasional occurrence of paraplegia reduces the patient to a pitiable state

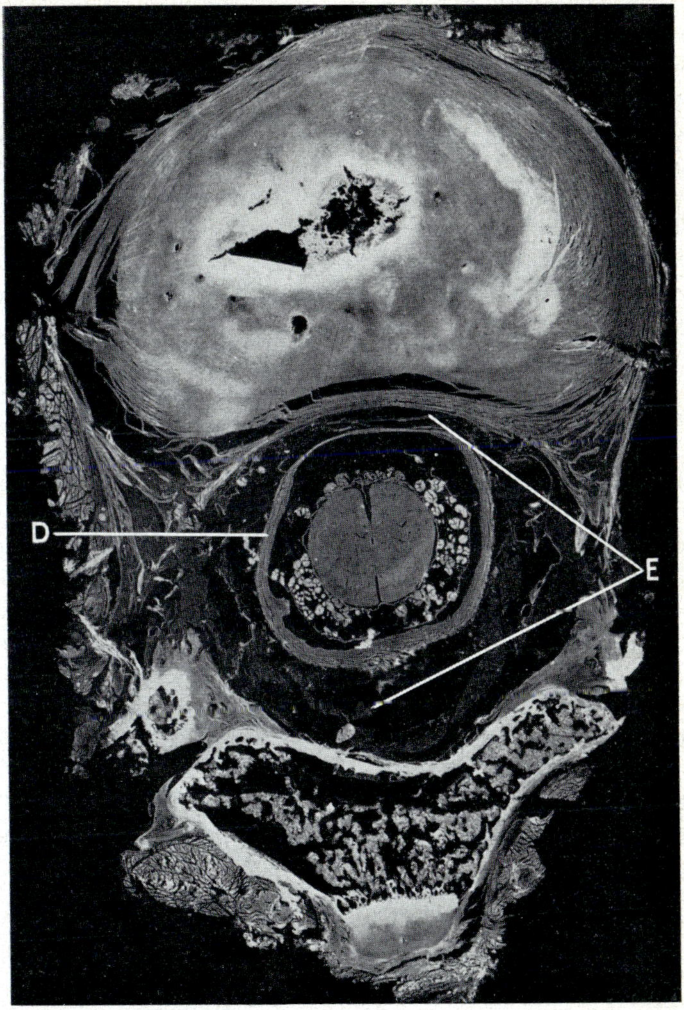

FIG. 7

Transverse section of spine between 1st and 2nd lumbar vertebrae. E is the epidural space and D the dura and arachnoid maters separating it from the subarachnoid space.

and has resulted in legal action being taken against the anaesthetist. The possibility of these complications has in this country at least persuaded most anaesthetists to reserve the technique for cases in which it is particularly indicated.

The complications of spinal analgesia have been widely investigated. The headache may be due to leakage of cerebrospinal fluid through the lumbar puncture and this can be minimised by using a fine needle. Paraplegia has been attributed to many things—infection, trauma, chemical irritation or the use of " unsuitable " solution. It may be due to the storage of ampoules of analgesic solution in antiseptic with subsequent seepage of the antiseptic into the solution. Some authorities, however, dispute this.

Many advantages of spinal analgesia without some of the complications may be obtained by extradural or epidural analgesia and this is now considered further.

Extradural or Epidural Analgesia (Figs. 6 and 7)

The nerves as they leave the subarachnoid space pass through the adjacent epidural or extradural space. This space is filled with fatty tissue and connects with the paravertebral spaces. By injecting analgesic solution into this space it is possible to obtain conditions identical to spinal blockade, namely good analgesia, sympathetic blockade and good muscular relaxation. Thus the risk of introducing infection into the subarachnoid space and the possibility of direct damage to the cord itself is eliminated. In addition as the arachnoid membrane is not punctured, headache is minimised. The main disadvantages of the technique are that the space is more difficult to identify than the subarachnoid space and the fat in it makes the spread of the solution less predictable. Thus the solution when injected may spread up or down the space or may leak out into the paravertebral space. Therefore for a given volume of solution it is less easy to predict accurately how far up in the space the solution will spread and therefore to what level analgesia will be produced. It should be pointed out also that paraplegia, though very rarely, has followed the use of this technique. Despite this it is favoured by many anaesthetists when subarachnoid anaesthesia might otherwise be indicated.

It is possible to pass a catheter into the extradural space and inject through it, at intervals, repeated doses of the analgesic solution. This enables analgesia to be continued into the post-operative period and by reducing post-operative pain deep breathing is facilitated and post-operative chest complications may be reduced. This method is also valuable in providing pain relief during labour (see p. 209).

GENERAL ANAESTHESIA

Anaesthesia involves the abolition of all sensation, touch, posture, temperature and pain and is a term normally reserved for states where the patient is unconscious. The mode of action of anaesthetic drugs is discussed later in this chapter but it serves at this point to mention that they act by producing a reversible depression of the central nervous system. In this way the patient is unconscious of painful impulses arriving from the periphery although it can be shown that under general anaesthesia the cortex is still receiving these stimuli.

Anaesthesia has three components, analgesia, hypnosis and muscular relaxation. Until less than 25 years ago it was common practice to produce all three by administration of potent inhalational agents such as ether, cyclopropane and more rarely chloroform. It is also possible to do so with the more modern potent anaesthetics such as halothane. However, with the introduction, by Griffiths of Montreal in 1942, of curare into anaesthetic practice, a new approach was made to the problem and Gray in Liverpool suggested the *triad* of anaesthesia as enumerated above. Since the unconscious patient does not " feel " pain in the normally accepted sense but rather shows reflex responses to it, " analgesia " is often replaced by " suppression of reflex activity " in the triad. It is in this context that the term " analgesia " is used when considering the unconscious patient in this work. By using small doses of specific drugs to produce separately hypnosis, analgesia and muscular relaxation it is possible to provide the appropriate combination for each patient.

Hypnosis

It is usual to induce hypnosis by intravenous injection of a short acting barbiturate, normally thiopentone or methohexitone or by propanidid. Alternatively one may induce unconsciousness with a gas such as nitrous oxide or cyclopropane or vapours such as halothane or ether. During anaesthesia hypnosis is maintained by inhalation of nitrous oxide and oxygen with, where necessary, addition of a more potent volatile agent such as halothane.

Analgesia

Adequate analgesia is often obtained by inhalation of nitrous oxide and oxygen but this may be supplemented by addition of a gas such as cyclopropane, the vapour of volatile agents, such as trichloroethylene, ether, halothane or methoxyflurane or by intravenous injection of a non-volatile analgesic such as pethidine. The choice of agent depends on many factors, including the use of diathermy which is incompatible with inflammable or explosive agents such as cyclopropane or ether and the use of adrenaline during operation which is incompatible with trichloroethylene, halothane or cyclopropane due to the high incidence of cardiac arrhythmias. Where a patient is breathing spontaneously one of the more potent agents is usually added to nitrous oxide and oxygen but where muscular relaxation is obtained by means of a specific relaxant and ventilation is controlled by the anaesthetist it is common practice to use only nitrous oxide and oxygen to provide analgesia.

Muscular Relaxation

Some degree of muscular relaxation is necessary for most operations. This may vary from simple relaxation of the forearm muscles during manipulation of a Colles' fracture to complete muscular paralysis for upper abdominal procedures or to produce apnoea during intra-thoracic operations. Until the early 1940s muscular relaxation was produced by the use of one of the more potent volatile anaesthetic agents, but the large quantities which were needed produced toxic effects on the liver and recourse was sometimes made to nerve blocks or to spinal or epidural techniques. However since the introduction of specific muscle relaxants into anaesthetic practice, most anaesthetists now use one of these drugs (p. 27).

MODE OF ACTION OF ANAESTHETIC DRUGS

General Anaesthesia

Anaesthesia is often defined as a reversible depression of the central nervous system. In some way oxygenation of the cerebral cells is temporarily interfered with and thus the patient becomes anaesthetised. It has been suggested that this depression of the brain is due to disturbances at the cell surfaces, to interference with enzyme systems within the cell or to physical changes within the cell. It may be produced by a wide variety of drugs—some hydrocarbons, the barbiturates and some alkaloids. A similar state may be brought about by inadequate oxygen tension in the inspired air, excess of carbon dioxide or possibly a very low level of carbon dioxide, by extreme cold and the controlled application of an electrical current. While the exact site of action of these several factors is in doubt, it now seems certain that a considerable part in the process is played by the reticular formation which is largely responsible for the maintenance of the conscious state. In the reticular formation there are many synapses and it is considered that anaesthetic agents act by interfering with synaptic transmission between cells rather than within the cell itself.

Anaesthetic agents must be soluble in water if they are to be dissolved in the plasma and carried to the brain. They must also be soluble in oil if they are to pass readily to the lipid tissue of the brain. Most anaesthetics therefore have a high oil/water solubility ratio.

Local Analgesic Drugs

It is known that the passage of impulses along nerves is associated with electrical changes. Sodium and potassium ions leave and enter the nerve during the different phases of conduction and this ionic migration takes place at the nodes of Ranvier, constrictions in the myelinated nerves at intervals of about 1 mm. It is the potential set up as these ions migrate which extends from one node to another and thus the impulse passes along the nerves. In some way, which is not fully understood, local analgesic drugs stabilise the nodal membrane to prevent ionic permeability and this interferes with the passage of impulses along the nerve and " blocks " the nerve.

Local analgesic solutions are stored for injection as water soluble salts, usually the hydrochloride. Such solutions are acid, having a low pH. When injected they come in contact with tissues which are alkaline (having a pH about 7·4) and this is sufficient to cause a reaction which liberates the base of the local analgesic. If an analgesic solution is injected into an infected area where the pH is low—down to about 5·6—the salt will fail to liberate base. This accounts for the failure of local analgesics to act in the presence of local infection.

The modes of action of analgesics and anaesthetics are extremely complicated and by no means established. The reader is referred to larger anaesthetic textbooks, or to works on pharmacology for detailed discussions on the subject.

CHAPTER II

PHARMACOLOGY

PHARMACOLOGY OF GENERAL ANAESTHETIC AGENTS

We can usefully describe the general anaesthetic agents under four headings.

1. The anaesthetic gases.
2. The volatile anaesthetic agents.
3. Non-anaesthetic gases used in anaesthesia.
4. Intravenous anaesthetics.

The Anaesthetic Gases

UPTAKE AND DISTRIBUTION OF ANAESTHETIC GASES. The gases and volatile agents used to produce general anaesthesia are absorbed on administration, transported to the cells of the central nervous system and other tissues of the body and finally excreted without any change taking place in their chemical composition. The different phases involved in the process are the inspiration of the mixture of anaesthetic gases and oxygen by the patient, the distribution of this mixture throughout the lungs and its diffusion across the alveolar capillary membrane. From this point the agent, in solution in the blood, returns to the heart from the lungs and is transported to the various tissues of the body and in particular to the brain. Here the anaesthetic agent diffuses through the capillary wall and finally enters the cells.

Many factors affect this process of absorption, transport and diffusion. Increase in the concentration of the anaesthetic gas or vapour, the alveolar ventilation and the partial pressure of the gas speed up the rate of absorption of the agent into the pulmonary capillary blood. The process of diffusion across the alveolar capillary membrane and the way in which the agent goes into solution in the blood depend on additional factors including the nature of the alveolar membrane, the solubility coefficient of the anaesthetic agent and the pulmonary blood flow. The rate at which the agent is transported to the tissues of the body will obviously vary with the cardiovascular state of the patient, including the cardiac output and systemic blood flow. Very vascular organs such as the brain, liver and kidneys will receive larger quantities of the anaesthetic drug and therefore the effect of the drug on these tissues will be earliest seen and most profound. The factors which control the diffusion of the drug into the cells themselves are not at all well understood.

HYPOXIA DURING ANAESTHESIA.—During anaesthesia either with a patient breathing spontaneously or where ventilation is controlled, some reduction in arterial oxygen tension is found where oxygen in atmospheric concentration (21 per cent.) is breathed.

A number of factors may cause this hypoxia, including an alteration in the ventilation/perfusion ratio in the lungs, where perfusion is greatest in the dependent parts and ventilation most effective in the upper zones. Depression of cardiac output may also lead to hypoxia as the desaturated blood from the coronary sinus and bronchial supply accounts for a higher proportion of the venous return. During controlled ventilation, unless high minute volumes are used, some areas of the lungs may be underventilated leading to arterio-venous " shunting " of blood.

While the mechanism is complex it is now widely accepted that the percentage of oxygen administered during anaesthesia should seldom be less than 30-33 per cent. as this has been shown to compensate for the other factors mentioned and to produce an arterial oxygen tension of at least 100 mm.Hg.

In circumstances where suitable apparatus or supplies of nitrous oxide and oxygen are not readily available, the use of air as a carrier gas for a volatile agent such as halothane or ether has been recommended. While this technique has proved valuable and in some circumstances will continue to do so, on the evidence quoted above its limitations must be borne in mind.

NITROUS OXIDE, the original " laughing gas ", is widely used. It is a weak anaesthetic and is rapidly eliminated from the body, mainly via the lungs, or redistributed thus ensuring quick recovery from anaesthesia. It is quite pleasant to inhale and is non-irritant and, provided it is given with an adequate concentration of oxygen, has no adverse effects on the vital organs. In addition post-operative vomiting and nausea are seldom experienced. As the gas is neither inflammable nor explosive it may be used safely in the presence of diathermy. It may also be used where it is intended to infiltrate adrenaline during the operation.

The mode of action of nitrous oxide is the subject of some dispute. There are those who claim that many of the signs of nitrous oxide/oxygen anaesthesia are those of hypoxia but its protagonists point out that anaesthesia may be induced with concentrations of oxygen which are equal to that breathed in the air. On the other hand it is claimed that nitrous oxide exerts its effects by oxygen displacement from the cerebral cells. If this is true some hypoxia is probably present.

In many robust patients it is difficult to maintain stable and adequate anaesthesia using nitrous oxide as the sole agent unless the oxygen concentration is reduced below 20 per cent. This being so it is now uncommon to administer the agent without some form of volatile adjuvant if anaesthesia is to be prolonged beyond a few minutes. Provided, however, care is taken to avoid hypoxia, nitrous oxide is indeed a safe anaesthetic within the above limitations. For most major surgical procedures anaesthesia is induced with an intravenous barbiturate, muscular relaxation produced with a specific muscle relaxant and analgesia obtained using nitrous oxide with 33 per cent. oxygen.

CYCLOPROPANE, in contrast to nitrous oxide, is a potent anaesthetic agent. It is non-irritant but not so pleasant to inhale as nitrous oxide. It is highly explosive and cannot be used in the presence of diathermy and infiltration of adrenaline should not be permitted during cyclopropane anaesthesia lest fatal cardiac arrhythmias occur. Even without the injection of adrenaline cardiac arrhythmias are not uncommon. The drug is a powerful respiratory depressant and if carbon dioxide accumulates cardiac arrhythmias develop. It may be given with very high concentrations of oxygen, up to 90 per cent., and was a popular anaesthetic agent for poor risk cases. As it is expensive it is normally used in a closed circuit. The increasing use of diathermy has rendered cyclopropane less popular and the introduction of halothane has removed many of the indications for its use. For rapid induction of anaesthesia in children, in outpatients and in dental anaesthesia cyclopropane is still used.

The Volatile Anaesthetic Agents

ETHER (diethyl ether) was for many years the most widely used of the volatile anaesthetic agents. Given either by the open drop method or in conjunction with nitrous oxide and oxygen, it has been used in all types of patients. Ether vapour is irritating and when inhaled may produce coughing, breath holding and laryngeal spasm. Secretions are increased and if atropine is not given may be troublesome. These very properties, however, tend to increase its safety since, although induction of anaesthesia may be slow, it is difficult to give an overdose of the drug. Even when respiratory arrest has occurred, provided controlled ventilation with oxygen is instituted, acute circulatory failure will not occur. With chloroform circulatory collapse may actually precede respiratory failure. If the anaesthetist takes time with his induction, fairly adequate muscular relaxation can be obtained for abdominal surgical procedures. With suitable vaporisers it may be used as the sole anaesthetic where other anaesthetic agents and apparatus are not available.

Ether is, however, inflammable and explosive and the increasing use of diathermy has reduced its use in many surgical centres. In addition it is associated with a fairly high percentage of post-operative nausea and vomiting (up to 50 per cent.) and the vapour is excreted by the lungs for some time post-operatively. It has been blamed for a high incidence of post-operative chest complications but it is now generally accepted that the incidence of " post-operative chests " is unrelated to the anaesthetic used.

DIVINYL ETHER is a more potent agent than diethyl ether. It is expensive and because of this and its hepatotoxicity is used as a rule either for short operations or for induction of anaesthesia. It is less irritant to inhale than ether, nausea and vomiting after short administrations are rare and recovery of consciousness is fairly rapid. The agent is considered to be four times as potent as ether and respiratory arrest is fairly easily produced.

A mixture containing divinyl (25 per cent.) and diethyl ether (75 per cent.) known as *Vinesthene Anaesthetic Mixture* was popular for short operations as it possessed the advantages of both agents.

ETHYL CHLORIDE, which was a popular drug for inducing anaesthesia before proceeding to ether, or for short operations, is seldom used today. It is a very potent agent indeed and very little more than the normal induction dose will produce cardiovascular and respiratory collapse. In addition laryngeal spasm and spasm of the masseters is not uncommon. Even before the introduction of halothane, ethyl chloride had largely been replaced by divinyl ether.

CHLOROFORM has probably been one of the most controversial anaesthetic agents. It is a very powerful anaesthetic, is relatively non-irritant and deep anaesthesia may be produced fairly easily with it. It has, however, serious effects on the cardiovascular system and has been responsible for cardiac arrest either by direct vagal inhibition or by producing ventricular fibrillation or by direct depression of the myocardium. Post-operative nausea and vomiting are said to occur in up to 50 per cent. of cases and liver damage in varying degree occurs. Its protagonists claim that used as halothane is now used, in known concentrations with adequate oxygen and by trained anaesthetists, it has much to commend it, being very much cheaper than halothane. However this claim has not been widely accepted and chloroform is seldom if ever used in anaesthetic practice nowadays. Diminishing numbers of practitioners use it for domiciliary obstetrics where apparatus for more sophisticated anaesthesia is unavailable.

TRICHLOROETHYLENE (TRILENE) is an anaesthetic said to resemble chloroform in some of its effects. It is however much less depressant and much safer. It is a good analgesic but a poor relaxant. Cardiac arrhythmias occur during administration of Trilene and occasionally cardiac arrest also. Trilene must not be used in a closed circuit as it reacts with soda lime forming toxic products. It is suitable only for producing light levels of anaesthesia and if pushed to greater depth a tachypnoea develops which interferes with adequate ventilation. In addition if Trilene in high concentration has been given for a prolonged period, recovery is very slow and may be accompanied by considerable nausea or vomiting. The agent is still widely used for producing analgesia in obstetrics, being used in temperature compensated vaporisers such as the Emotril or

Tecota which give a low concentration of the drug under all circumstances. Trilene should not be used with adrenaline infiltration lest arrhythmias be converted to ventricular fibrillation. It is, however, non-inflammable and can be used in the presence of diathermy. In many centres it has been replaced by the much more potent halothane.

HALOTHANE (FLUOTHANE). This agent, since its introduction, has achieved wide popularity despite its great potency and the fact that it is very expensive. It is a clear heavy liquid which, though it resembles chloroform in some ways, lacks many of the disadvantages of chloroform.

It is non-irritant to inhale and though having a rather sickly smell is considered by many to be not unpleasant. It is a very powerful agent, being one and a half times as potent as chloroform and about five times as potent as diethyl ether. As it is non-irritant, the depth of anaesthesia can be rapidly altered by the skilled anaesthetist. Provided large quantities of the drug have not been given over a long period, recovery is fairly rapid and nausea and vomiting are less than after ether or chloroform or indeed after cyclopropane anaesthesia. Bleeding may be reduced during operation as there is a depression of cardiac output and a fall in blood pressure. The vapour is not inflammable or explosive and may be used in the presence of diathermy. Muscular relaxation can be produced but normally only by giving high concentrations of the drug which reduce the blood pressure and depress respiration beyond what is considered desirable. It can rapidly lead to severe respiratory and cardiovascular depression and in addition it produces marked uterine relaxation. In obstetric cases, therefore, it is usually avoided lest haemorrhage follow delivery of the baby. Occasionally it is, however, used in obstetric cases to produce the relaxation of the uterus required for external version. In contrast to trichloroethylene it is a poor analgesic in low concentration.

Halothane, when used with nitrous oxide and oxygen, is a very useful anaesthetic for many purposes. It is used widely in this way but its use as the sole anaesthetic for producing muscular relaxation in major surgery is restricted to a few enthusiasts. In the hands of the expert it is a very valuable drug and has displaced many or most of the other volatile agents as the supplement to nitrous oxide and oxygen. While it appears simple to use, the safety margin is very small and overdosage may be readily produced. Warning signs are tachypnoea, bradycardia and fall in blood pressure. One cynical anaesthetist has stated that fully developed halothane anaesthesia is associated with the figure 50. A blood pressure of 50, a respiratory rate of 50 and a heart rate of 50!

METHOXYFLURANE is a halogenated ether with a high boiling point (104·6° C) and is therefore slow to vaporise. Induction of anaesthesia and recovery time are therefore both prolonged. The vapour is compatible with soda lime but methoxyflurane must be used cautiously when adrenaline infiltration is contemplated. It is non-inflammable in the concentrations which can be produced in clinical practice (up to 4 per cent.). Deep anaesthesia with methoxyflurane may cause hypotension and very slow recovery to full consciousness. It is however an effective analgesic in low concentrations (0·5 per cent.) and is most commonly used as such in labour (see p. 207) or as a supplement to nitrous oxide-oxygen anaesthesia for prolonged surgery.

The Non-anaesthetic Gases Associated with Anaesthesia

CARBON DIOXIDE has anaesthetic properties of its own when used in concentrations in excess of 30 per cent. but it is not for this reason that it is normally used in anaesthetic practice. It is a respiratory stimulant increasing both the rate and depth of respiration when added to the gas mixtures inhaled. It may be added directly to the mixture from a cylinder which is normally kept on the anaesthetic machine or may be allowed to accumulate in the anaesthetic circuit by reducing the flow of gases below the patient's minute volume and closing the valve so that rebreathing takes place. Its use as a respiratory stimulant should however be restricted because it must be remembered that in most cases where respiration is depressed and a stimulant is needed there is already retention of carbon dioxide. There is little point therefore in " adding thy sum of more to that which hath too much ".

The use of carbon dioxide is therefore strictly limited. It may be added during induction of anaesthesia, particularly with ether or other irritant vapours, so that respiration is stimulated and induction time reduced. During upper abdominal surgery it may occasionally be given to relieve hiccough, or at the end of a long operation where hyperventilation has been practised and it is known that the tension of carbon dioxide in the blood is reduced, a small amount may be added to the gas mixture for a very limited period.

OXYGEN is given in all anaesthetic techniques. It may be inhaled in air or may be added to the anaesthetic mixtures, in atmospheric concentration, that is about 20 per cent., but usually in excess of this (see page 14). The use of cyclopropane or halothane allows the administration of high concentrations, up to 90 per cent., of oxygen and this method is practised by some anaesthetists. While breathing 100 per cent. oxygen initially depresses respiration, before stimulating it, probably through the chemoreceptors, during anaesthesia the stimulant effect is seldom seen as the anaesthetic agents given with high concentrations of oxygen are themselves respiratory depressants. High concentrations of oxygen decrease the heart rate and reduce cardiac output and blood pressure. In addition, the agents which are normally given with high concentrations of oxygen depress the heart rate and blood pressure.

There are adverse effects to be found from breathing high concentrations of oxygen. Nitrogen is washed out from the alveoli and as oxygen is rapidly absorbed, patchy atelectasis may occur. Further, by supplying excess oxygen with minimal respiratory effort, respiration becomes depressed and this leads to carbon dioxide retention. As a high concentration of oxygen is given the patient does not become cyanosed until a very late stage and often because the patient retains his colour and is a " nice pink colour " the onlooker may not realise that respiratory depression is present.

More recently oxygen has been used at higher than atmospheric pressure in a variety of circumstances. This technique enables the tension in the plasma to be raised several times and thus more oxygen is easily available to the tissues. This is valuable in the treatment of patients with carbon monoxide poisoning, barbiturate poisoning, various cardiovascular diseases and anaerobic infections such as gas gangrene. It is considered further in Chapter X.

Intravenous Anaesthetic Agents

THIOPENTONE SODIUM is the sulphur analogue of pentobarbitone. It is supplied as a yellowish powder with an ampoule or bottle of sterile water sufficient to make up either a 5 per cent. or a 2·5 per cent. solution. As the yellow powder contains 6 per cent. sodium carbonate to stop the formation of the insoluble thiopentone acid, the solution has a high pH (10·4 - 10·6). This solution is prepared immediately before use as it is relatively unstable and is not normally kept for longer than 24 to 48 hours. Thiopentone like other barbiturates causes sedation and induces sleep but has no analgesic activity and it has been shown in small doses to have an antanalgesic effect. This is responsible for some of the post-operative restlessness which is found in patients where anaesthesia has been induced with thiopentone and pain is prominent after operation. For this reason also it is unsatisfactory to use thiopentone as the sole anaesthetic in any but the shortest procedures.

The drug depresses the respiratory centre and after a deep breath or even a yawn, respiration is reduced, mainly in amplitude. Apnoea may supervene for a few moments then breathing restarts, still shallow and regular. This shallow respiration, however, is easily increased in amplitude by any surgical stimulus and indeed by further anaesthetic manipulations such as subsequent venepuncture.

A fall in blood pressure usually accompanies the injection of thiopentone though this may be minimised by slow steady injection. It is largely due to vasodilatation of the peripheral vascular bed and is as a rule transient provided only small doses of the drug have been given.

Another effect which is of importance in anaesthetic practice is that the autonomic nervous system is depressed, the sympathetic more than the parasympathetic. This results in relative parasympathetic overactivity which may give rise to laryngeal spasm, bronchospasm, coughing and bucking during the induction of anaesthesia.

Recovery from a single " sleep dose " of thiopentone is rapid, partly due to the breakdown of the drug in the liver and partly due to redistribution in the body. After recovery of consciousness the redistributed drug is gradually fed back into the blood and then broken down. Barbiturate in small quantities can be detected in the blood up to 24 hours after administration and it is for this reason that it is dangerous for the out-patient to drive a car soon after recovery or to consume other drugs or alcohol. The breakdown products are excreted via the kidney and in patients with a high blood urea the drug should be used with extreme caution.

The solution of thiopentone is extremely alkaline (pH 10·4-10·6); if it is injected extravenously, in the subcutaneous tissues or worse still into an artery, severe damage may result. Accidental injection into the subcutaneous tissues may result in abscess formation with an indolent ulcer developing later, while intra-arterial injection results in severe vascular spasm and thrombosis and possibly gangrene of the affected part. These complications are dealt with when considering intravenous induction of anaesthesia.

Despite the introduction of many more modern intravenous anaesthetic agents, thiopentone is still the agent most widely used to induce anaesthesia.

METHOHEXITONE SODIUM. This drug is one of the many which have been introduced in an attempt to avoid some of the undesirable effects of thiopentone. It is used in 1 per cent. solution with a pH of 11·1. The recovery time is claimed to be shorter than after thiopentone and the recovery to be more complete, that is when the patient wakens up he does so with very little in the way of " hangover " effect. The out-patient is therefore able to leave the surgery or to go home sooner and more safely. Some patients who receive injections of methohexitone intravenously may complain of pain at the site of injection or along the course of the vein during the injection despite the fact that the needle is correctly positioned within the vein.

Some workers have found a high incidence of hiccough and of muscular movements and twitching following the administration of methohexitone. There is considerable disagreement as to how often this occurs but it does so more often than after thiopentone. It may be that this incidence of muscular movement can be diminished by giving an analgesic premedication such as pethidine. Many anaesthetists have found the drug useful in dental practice and in outpatient anaesthetic work, but it has not so far displaced thiopentone from routine theatre work.

PROPANIDID (EPONTOL). Propanidid, a non-barbiturate eugenol derivative, is now frequently used as an induction agent before proceeding to inhalational anaesthesia. The drug is roughly equipotent with thiopentone but is poorly soluble in water and is dissolved in an oily base, which makes a very viscid solution. After injection of a single dose of 5 - 7 mg./Kg. the patient hyperventilates and loses consciousness for a period of 3 - 5 minutes. Recovery is more rapid and complete than after thiopentone and unlike the barbiturates it is rapidly broken down without appreciable redistribution in the body.

The drug potentiates the neuromuscular blocking action of suxamethonium but the incidence of post-operative muscle pains after suxamethonium is reduced.

Propanidid is most useful in out-patient anaesthesia.

STEROID ANAESTHETICS. For some years hydroxydione, a steroid compound, has been used as an anaesthetic agent. Unlike the barbiturates, in low concentrations it has analgesic properties. Onset of action is slower than with the barbiturates but laryngeal activity is reduced and less respiratory and cardiovascular depression are normally produced.

The main disadvantage of the drug is its irritant action on vein walls causing an unacceptably high incidence of post-operative venous thrombosis.

Other steroid derivatives, also devoid of hormonal activity, are being studied and may lead to a wider use of this interesting group of drugs.

KETAMINE. This drug, a powerful analgesic, may be given intravenously and produces profound analgesia with a state of dissociation from the environment and sometimes unconsciousness, usually with inhibition of protective reflexes. Despite the advantages claimed for this agent, its use is limited by the occurrence of systemic hypertension after administration and the high incidence of vivid dreams or hallucinations experienced during recovery.

DIAZEPAM (Valium). This drug, a benzodiazepine, used principally as a tranquilliser, has been used by intravenous injection to induce anaesthesia. It is claimed that it produces less respiratory and circulatory depression than the barbiturates. On some occasions, even using fairly large doses, the patients do not lose consciousness but readily accept an inhalational induction of anaesthesia. Diazepam has muscle relaxant properties which make it valuable in controlling convulsions. It seems however unlikely to supplant the more established agents such as thiopentone for routine induction of anaesthesia.

NEUROLEPTANALGESIA. The drugs used in this technique comprise:

1. " Neuroleptic " drugs which produce a state of dissociation—usually a pleasant sensation but sometimes associated with acute anxiety. Such drugs include haloperidol, dehydrobenzperidol (droperidol) and spiroperidol. They are potent anti-emetic agents, depressing the chemoreceptor trigger zone in the mid brain. Unfortunately, they may also cause Parkinsonian tremors.

2. Potent analgesics such as fentanyl and phenoperidine which, in addition to providing analgesia, in common with other similar drugs such as pethidine, may cause nausea, vomiting and respiratory depression.

Mixtures of the drugs, one from each group, may be used to induce a state of unconsciousness with profound analgesia Anaesthesia is maintained with nitrous oxide and oxygen and where required a muscle relaxant drug (see also p. 101). While it is claimed that a stable blood pressure and some protection from shock is provided by this combination of drugs, the patient may be drowsy though rousable for a considerable period post-operatively.

PHARMACOLOGY OF PREMEDICANT AGENTS

Sedatives

THE OPIATES. Morphine and allied drugs are still widely used in premedication today despite the many other drugs which are available. They produce analgesia, psychic sedation and a state of euphoria which is very welcome before an operation. The opiates are non-irritant solutions and may be injected subcutaneously or intramuscularly. Their main disadvantages are that they produce a high incidence of post-operative vomiting, 30-40 per cent., and are respiratory depressants. In addition they increase parasympathetic activity predisposing to laryngeal spasm and possibly bronchospasm. It has been suggested that they should not be used in asthmatic patients for this reason.

Morphine sulphate is normally given in a dose of 1·5 mg. per stone to a maximum of 15 mg. Papaveretum, containing morphine plus the other alkaloids of opium, is usually administered in a dose of 2 mg. per stone to a maximum of 20 mg. Papaveretum is considered less liable to produce nausea and vomiting than morphine sulphate although this is perhaps doubtful. Many of the disadvantages of the opiates are found when in fact too large a dose is given for a particular patient. It has been well said that there is a correct dose of morphine for every patient.

PETHIDINE HYDROCHLORIDE was introduced as a substitute for morphine. It was claimed to produce less respiratory depression and less nausea and vomiting than the opiates. Recent work has cast some doubt on each of these claims. In addition pethidine is a poorer sedative and produces less euphoria than the opiates. Given in equi-analgesic dosage the side-effects are probably similar to those found after the use of morphine and the sedative properties are much less (morphine 10 mg.≡pethidine 60-65 mg.).

Pethidine is claimed to have a relaxant effect on the bronchi and may be useful in cases where bronchospasm is present or suspected. In addition it is useful in producing dilatation of the cervix in labour and is widely used in obstetric practice for this reason.

The use of analgesic agents in premedication has been frequently questioned. It is claimed that when administered to pain-free anxious patients they frequently fail to relieve anxiety and produce a state of confusion or dysphoria. It is also claimed that if narcotics are omitted from premedication but given during or after anaesthesia, when the patient is in pain, the incidence of emetic sequelae is reduced. Thus, attention has been directed towards other groups of drugs.

THE HYPNOTICS. Barbiturate and other hypnotic drugs may be used to produce a state of tranquillity before operation. While these drugs are not analgesics, relief of anxiety *per se* frequently reduces the severity of post-operative pain and a reduction in the dosage of analgesics may be achieved. Alternatively, a smaller dose of analgesic may be combined with a sedative drug as premedication. In this way better pre-operative sedation and less post-operative sickness is produced.

THE PHENOTHIAZINES. These drugs like the hypnotics have been used to allay pre-operative anxiety. Many of the group have also anti-emetic properties. As in the case of the hypnotics, few phenothiazines have any analgesic properties but they may usefully be combined with a small dose of an analgesic. A popular combination is the mixture of pethidine with promethazine (Phenergan).

The phenothiazines tend to produce hypotension, particularly in combination with some anaesthetic agents. Similarly, post-operative drowsiness may be prolonged. This has tended to limit their use.

THE BENZODIAZEPINES. This group of drugs, including chlordiazepoxide (Librium) and diazepam (Valium), has been widely used in premedication either orally or by injection as they have been shown to possess specific anti-anxiety properties. Small doses of these drugs may be given from the time of admission to hospital until shortly before operation.

When using any of these sedative non-analgesic drugs as premedication in patients undergoing operations known to produce considerable post-operative pain, administration of small doses of an analgesic towards the end of operation is valuable. Alternatively, adequate arrangements must be available to ensure that post-operative analgesics are administered as soon as they are required.

Atropine and Hyoscine

One or other of these drugs is often given before an anaesthetic in order to minimise the parasympathetic over-activity which may be found during the anaesthetic itself. While the use of non-irritant drugs reduces the need for these belladonna derivatives, they are still widely employed.

They have some common actions. Both depress secretions from the salivary glands and from the mucous glands in the bronchial tree. In addition they antagonise the muscarinic effects of acetylcholine. The pupil is dilated, the bronchial musculature is relaxed and a slight increase in respiratory dead-space may therefore result. The tone and peristalsis in the alimentary tract are diminished.

The two drugs however differ in certain respects.

ATROPINE is more effective in blocking the muscarinic effects on the heart. Thus a mild tachycardia follows its administration and there is less response to the administration of such drugs as neostigmine or halothane which would otherwise cause a bradycardia. It has however no sedative effect and in fact increases the basal metabolic rate and stimulates the medulla and higher centres.

HYOSCINE (Scopolamine) differs in that it produces a depression of the central nervous system causing drowsiness, sleep and amnesia. These effects are valuable in premedication and the drug is often combined with an opiate or pethidine. The action on the heart and bronchial musculature is weaker than that of atropine and the heart indeed may be slightly slowed after administration of hyoscine. However the drying effect of the drug is greater than atropine and this may prove valuable when irritant agents are employed.

Hyoscine has been shown to have a beneficial effect in reducing the incidence of travel sickness, and it was extensively used for this purpose during the war. It is also of value in minimising post-operative vomiting. The main disadvantage of the drug is that, particularly in older people, it may cause confusion and restlessness which may be very distressing for the patient and his attendants.

DOSAGE. Atropine is normally given in a dose of 0·3-1·2 mg. and hyoscine in a dose of 0·4-0·6 mg.

PHARMACOLOGY OF MUSCLE RELAXANT AGENTS

As the name implies these drugs specifically relax striated muscle but have no effect on consciousness. They can be divided into two categories according to their action at the neuromuscular junction. The latter is shown diagrammatically in Figure 8. When a stimulus passes down a nerve, acetylcholine is released at the neuromuscular junction and this triggers off the contraction of the muscle. The acetylcholine is broken down by cholinesterase and the muscle returns to its resting state.

The Competitive or Non-depolarising Relaxants

CURARE was the first muscle relaxant to be introduced into anaesthetic practice and is still refined from the extracts of plants brought from South America. The South American Indians used this agent as an arrow poison and their victims were paralysed and died from asphyxia. *d*-tubocurarine is the muscle relaxant of choice in many centres. It is administered in a solution containing 10 mg. per ml. and the normal dose required to produce complete muscular relaxation is about 30 mg. Paralysis of all muscles develops in about three minutes and adequate time must be allowed for the drug to act. It is not preceded by any stimulation of the muscles but is accompanied by a slow gradual depression of respiration which finally

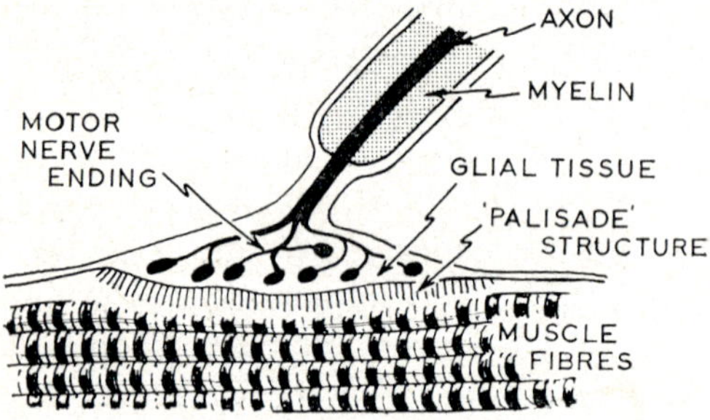

FIG. 8
The myoneural junction: The "palisade" structure is the site at which acetylcholine, released from the motor nerve endings, acts upon the muscle fibres to cause contraction.

ceases. In the dosage used in clinical practice, that is 30 to 60 mg. and even in slightly greater dosage, possibly up to 80 mg., few effects are seen apart from paralysis of the neuromuscular junction. However with larger doses or perhaps in some sensitive individuals, ganglionic blockade may be caused and this is associated with a fall in blood pressure. It is also claimed that with the larger doses histamine release may take place and an asthmatic type of reaction may be found. These effects are rarely seen, however, and are not considered contra-indications to the use of the drug.

GALLAMINE TRIETHIODIDE (Flaxedil) is a synthetic agent which has a similar action to that of curare, that is, it is a non-depolarising blocker. Being synthesised in this country, it is cheaper than tubocurarine though less potent (120 mg. equal to about 30 mg. of curare). In addition to producing paralysis at the neuromuscular junction, it causes tachycardia but has little or no effect on the blood pressure and is less liable to produce histamine release than is curare. As a high percentage of the drug is excreted by the kidneys its use is contra-indicated in the presence of impaired renal function.

The effect of curare lasts from 30 to 40 minutes while gallamine acts for 20 to 30 minutes.

ALCURONIUM (Alloferin) is a non-depolarising muscle relaxant said to be about twice as potent as *d*-tubocurarine but with otherwise similar properties.

PANCURONIUM BROMIDE (Pavulon) is also a non-depolarising muscle relaxant, five to six times more potent than d-tubocurarine and, like this agent and alcuronium, does not produce tachycardia. It produces no hypotension in contrast to curare and may be used in conjunction with halothane with less risk of causing a marked fall in blood pressure.

NEOSTIGMINE (Prostigmin) which is an anticholinesterase, allows the concentration of acetylcholine to rise and is therefore an antagonist to gallamine, curare, alcuronium or pancuronium.

It must be stressed that the muscle relaxants have no analgesic or anaesthetic properties. It is therefore essential that the patients are supplied with an analgesic and anaesthetic mixture and that ventilation is maintained by artificial means.

The Depolarising Relaxants

SUXAMETHONIUM CHLORIDE (Scoline) and SUXETHONIUM BROMIDE (Brevidil E) are depolarising agents with an action similar to that of acetylcholine. They produce initial muscle twitching and fasciculation followed by paralysis which lasts from two to four minutes. Following the administration of suxamethonium there is a transient rise in blood pressure and often a slowing of the heart which is particularly noticeable with second and subsequent injections of the drug. It has been reported that in some cases the heart stopped for a period of up to seven seconds. These effects can be minimised by the intravenous administration of atropine prior to the induction of anaesthesia.

Suxamethonium and suxethonium are hydrolysed in the blood by pseudocholinesterase found in the plasma. In some cases this enzyme may be atypical or may be abnormally low in concentration, and the effect of suxamethonium may be prolonged for a considerable period. There is no antagonist to these depolarising relaxants except fresh plasma which contains pseudocholinesterase.

DECAMETHONIUM IODIDE (C10) has been used as a depolarising relaxant, its action lasting about 15 minutes. Again however it has no antagonist and is not widely used today, as the competitive blocking agents with similar duration of action are preferred.

PHARMACOLOGY OF VASOPRESSOR DRUGS

There is occasionally a need to restore a low blood pressure to a more normal level. The hypotension may have been deliberately induced to provide a bloodless surgical field but the anaesthetist may wish to raise the blood pressure during, or at the end of, the surgical procedure. The administration of a suitable dose of vasopressor drug assists the anaesthetist to control the pressure at will. In other circumstances profound and dangerous hypotension may follow excessive blood loss and a vasopressor may have to be given to restore the blood pressure while a blood transfusion is set up. This stop-gap procedure is a temporary measure and not a substitute for restoring a normal blood volume.

Although a great number of vasopressor drugs are currently available, the anaesthetist generally requires to use only one of a small number of these drugs. It is important to bear in mind certain general considerations before using these drugs.

TACHYPHYLAXIS is a phenomenon encountered with most vasopressors, i.e. bigger doses or more frequent doses of the drug have to be given to achieve the same effect, if the drug has to be administered over a long period of time. The *mode of action* of the individual drug is important since it may act on the heart or directly on the blood vessels, or on both. *Adrenaline,* and the vasopressor group which have an adrenaline-like action, the *sympathomimetic amines,* must not be given in the presence of chloroform, cyclopropane, or trichloroethylene. Cardiac arrhythmias and ventricular fibrillation can result when this point is forgotten.

If the patient has been receiving *phenothiazine drugs* prior to operation, the action of the vasopressor drugs may be interfered with and a poor response may follow a normal dose of the drug. Hypotension has actually followed the administration of noradrenaline to a patient previously treated with chlorpromazine. Vasopressor drugs may also fail to act in patients whose hypotension is a result of adrenal hypofunction. The intravenous administration of hydrocortisone hemisuccinate (100 mg.) usually raises the blood pressure in these cases.

Vasopressors must be used with extreme caution in patients with cardiovascular disease or thyrotoxicosis.

The following are some of the more useful drugs in anaesthetic practice.

Methyl-amphetamine (Methedrine)

This drug is a sympathomimetic amine. It produces its pressor effect by acting centrally to increase the rate and force of contraction of the heart, and it also has a powerful peripheral vasoconstrictor effect. This drug stimulates the central nervous system, like its close relative amphetamine, and a lightly anaesthetised patient may awaken following its use. The drug has a long action and tachyphylaxis is not usually marked.

DOSE: 15-30 mg. intramuscularly or 5-10 mg. intravenously.

Because of the widespread abuse of amphetamines by addicts, this drug is now seldom used as other vasopressors with no addiction liability are available.

Methoxamine (Vasoxyl, Vasoxine)

This is a synthetic drug with a powerful peripheral vasoconstrictor action. It does not cause stimulation of the central nervous system. Bradycardia may be observed. Methoxamine is very useful in anaesthetic practice since it is compatible with cyclopropane and halothane. The drug has an action of about one hour and its effect can be observed within two minutes of intravenous injection.

DOSE: 5-15 mg. intramuscularly or 2 mg. intravenously.

Metaraminol (Aramine)

This is a potent vasopressor with a prolonged duration of action. Although it appears to be relatively free from the danger of causing cardiac arrhythmias, nevertheless it is a sympathomimetic amine and should not be used during trichloroethylene, halothane or cyclopropane anaesthesia.

DOSE: 2-10 mg. intramuscularly or subcutaneously.

For intravenous use 15-100 mg. may be added to 500 ml. sodium chloride or 5 per cent. dextrose in water. See Chapter VI.

l-noradrenaline (Levophed)

Adrenaline itself is rarely used by anaesthetists to raise the blood pressure, mainly because of its violent effect and comparatively short duration of action. Noradrenaline is preferred to adrenaline but is used only as a last resort, when other safer vasopressors have failed. The drug is a powerful peripheral vasoconstrictor and highly irritant should any leak into the tissues at the site of the venepuncture (p. 265). Tachyphylaxis is very common and there is sometimes difficulty in weaning the patient from the drug after it has been used for a long time. Adrenaline has been mentioned as being dangerous when used with certain anaesthetic agents and it has been claimed that noradrenaline is safer under these circumstances, particularly if used in a dilution of not more than 1:250,000.

DOSE: 2 ml. of the 1:1,000 solution of noradrenaline is usually added to 500 ml. of 5 per cent. dextrose in water and given slowly as an intravenous infusion. The rate of administration is controlled according to the blood pressure response.

PHARMACOLOGY OF ADRENERGIC RECEPTOR BLOCKING DRUGS

Another group of drugs, the adrenergic receptor blockers, is worthy of the anaesthetist's attention. These drugs produce their effects by blocking the action of noradrenaline, the adrenergic transmitter substance, at the α and β receptor sites in the heart and blood vessels (Fig. 9A). Phenoxybenzamine and phentolamine, used in the diagnosis and pre-operative preparation of patients with phaeochromocytoma, act by competing with noradrenaline for the α receptor sites. Phenoxybenzamine may also be used in bacteraemic (endotoxic) shock to produce vasodilatation. Blood volume expanders are then administered and the metabolic acidosis corrected. The greatly improved tissue perfusion achieved contrasts markedly with the results which were obtained when vasopressors were used in this condition.

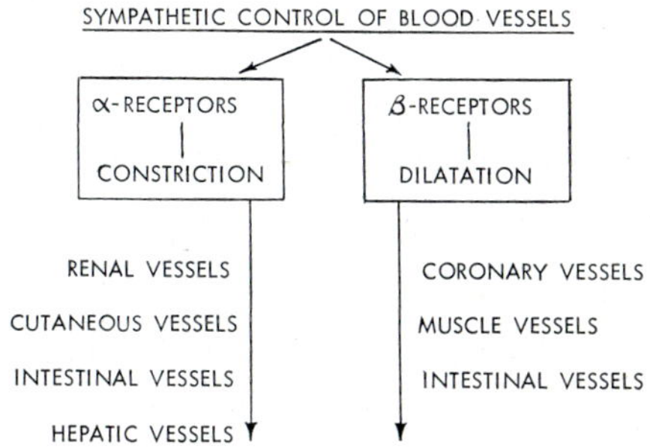

FIG. 9A

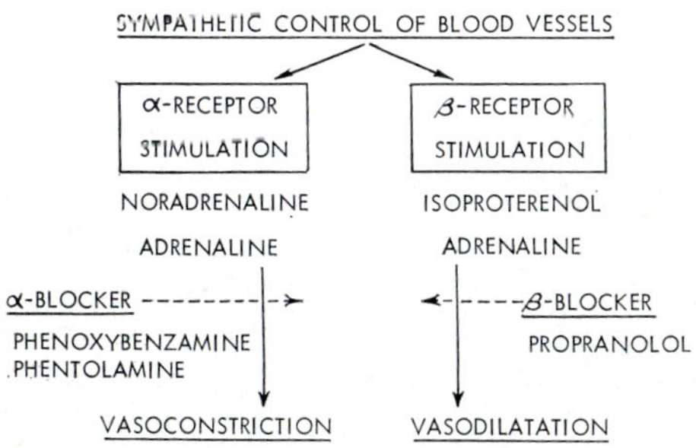

FIG. 9B

Propranolol, a β receptor blocker, used for the treatment of cardiac arrhythmias associated with an increased heart rate, does not block the vasoconstrictor pathways (Fig. 9B). It can be combined with an α receptor blocker to provide control of the hypertension associated with phaeochromocytoma. Propranolol may aggravate existing heart failure or even precipitate it and if signs of failure are present it should only be used if digitalis is already being given. Bradycardia and hypotension associated with its use, and probably due to vagal overaction, should be treated with intravenous atropine. The drug is contra-indicated in patients with bronchial asthma or bronchospasm.

Propranolol may be used in hypotensive anaesthesia in " resistant " patients whose blood pressure does not respond to the ganglion blocker drug being used and where tachycardia is a persistent feature. The drug produces a slowing of the heart rate and enables smaller doses of the ganglion blocking drug to be used.

DOSE: *Orally*: 10 to 20 mg. three times per day. *Intravenously*: The initial dose is 1 mg. injected over a period of one minute. This is repeated at intervals until a response is obtained. A total dose of 5 mg. should not be exceeded in the anaesthetised patient.

PHARMACOLOGY OF LOCAL ANALGESIC AGENTS

This subject is dealt with in Chapter XVI at page 223.

CHAPTER III

ANAESTHETIC MACHINES AND APPARATUS

While the early anaesthetics were given with the simplest of apparatus (Fig. 10), the modern anaesthetist uses what are to many people large, shiny and complicated machines. While at first sight these machines are indeed complicated they are, in fact, composed of five simple systems (Fig. 11).

1. A supply of compressed gases.
2. A method of reducing these gases to workable pressure.
3. A method of releasing and metering the gases.
4. A method of vaporising volatile anaesthetic agents.
5. A means of delivering the gases and vapours to the patient.

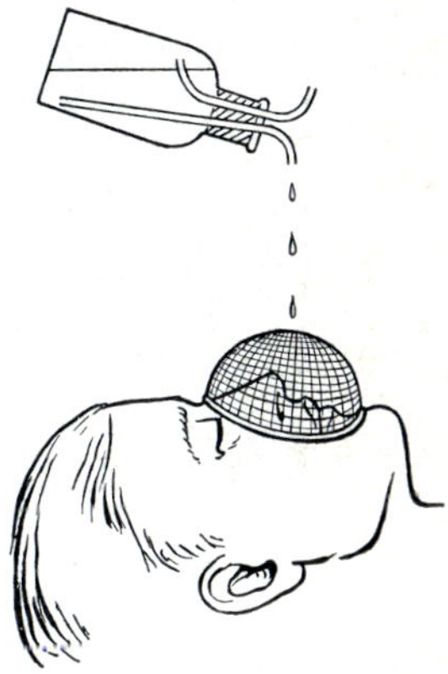

FIG. 10
Wire frame mask covered with gauze on which agent is dropped.

The Supply of Gases

This may take one of two forms. On most machines there is provision for two cylinders of nitrous oxide, two of oxygen, one of carbon dioxide and one

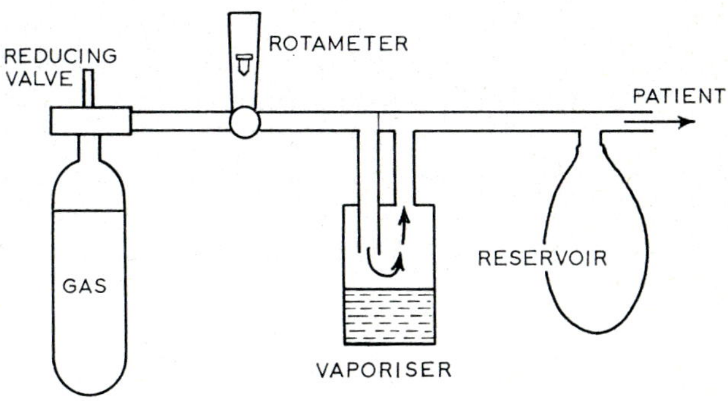

FIG. 11
Diagrammatic representation of the five components of a simple anaesthetic apparatus.

of cyclopropane. These cylinders may be used as the main supply of gases and the machine in this case is fairly mobile. It is customary to use one nitrous oxide cylinder and one oxygen cylinder at any one time, keeping the other two tightly closed and in reserve. In hospitals where considerable quantities of these gases are used, it is more economical to buy them in large cylinders which are stored at a convenient place some distance from the theatre and the gases are then piped to the theatres, connection being made between the end of the pipeline and the anaesthetic machine. Oxygen may be stored in liquid form and this is a further saving in cost. Even where the pipeline system is employed, however, at least one cylinder of each gas should be kept on the machine as a reserve in case of failure of the pipeline supply.

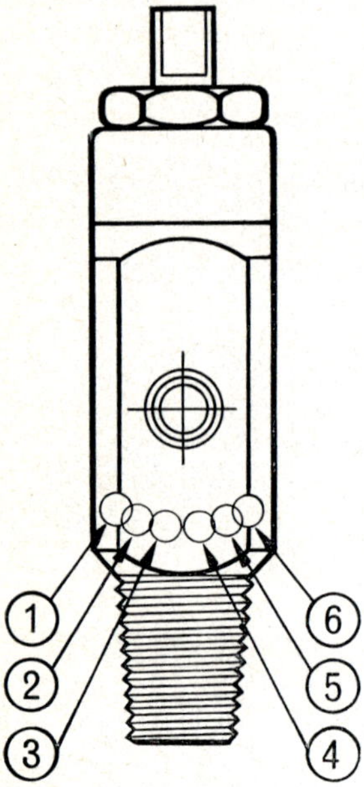

FIG. 12
This diagram shows how the holes on the cylinder neck are drilled on an arc. Only two holes are found on each cylinder *e.g.*:
2 & 5 on oxygen cylinders
3 & 5 on nitrous oxide cylinders
3 & 6 on cyclopropane cylinders.

The cylinders are readily identifiable, each being painted in a distinctive colour—oxygen being black with white shoulders, nitrous oxide blue, cyclopropane orange and carbon dioxide grey. In addition the name of the gas is printed on the cylinder as is the chemical symbol. A further safeguard against connecting a cylinder to the wrong reducing valve is that in the head of the cylinder, beside the port out of which the gas flows, two small holes are drilled in positions specific for each gas (Fig. 12). These match two pins on the reducing valve.

In addition to identifying the cylinders containing a particular gas, it is important to know how much of the gas each cylinder contains. In the case of oxygen, the reducing valve connected to the cylinder has attached to it a pressure gauge and the contents of the cylinder can be measured by estimating the pressure. A full cylinder contains gas at a pressure of approximately 2,000 lb./sq. in. and as the volume of gas in the cylinder falls the pressure is proportionately reduced. A device is available which gives visual and audible warning when the oxygen cylinder is empty. Nitrous oxide and carbon dioxide are however stored as liquids and the pressure above the liquid remains the same until very little liquid remains in the cylinder (Fig. 13). Because of this a pressure gauge would only be of value to the anaesthetist at this stage.

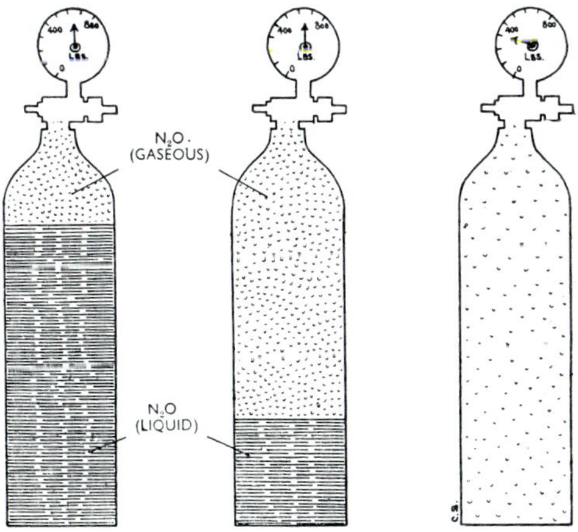

FIG. 13
Pressure of N_2O as recorded by gauge remains constant until very little liquid remains in the cylinder.

This indication is however better than none and in some modern anaesthetic machines, the pressure gauge may be incorporated in the reducing valve for use with nitrous oxide. The normal method of ascertaining how much nitrous oxide remains in the cylinder, however, is to weigh the cylinder and by subtracting the tare weight of the cylinder, which is embossed on the neck, one can determine how much nitrous oxide is left in the cylinder (200 gallons of nitrous oxide weigh 60 oz.).

Clip-on labels are provided which may be attached to the reducing valve showing the words " full ", " in use " or " empty ". When a cylinder becomes empty it should be removed as soon as possible and be replaced with a full cylinder, failing which an " empty " label should be placed on the reducing valve. If this is not possible, it is wise to disconnect the reducing valve from the cylinder as a reminder that this cylinder must be replaced at the first opportunity.

When in theatre learn the layout of the suite, and find out where full cylinders of anaesthetic gases are kept. A full cylinder normally has a red cellophane wrapper covering the outlet port and if this is not in place the cylinder should be treated as empty until proved otherwise. Failure to replace empty cylinders is at best inconsiderate and may be frankly dangerous. It would be well if a notice was placed on each anaesthetic machine, ' Please leave this machine as you would wish to find it."

Reducing Valves

The pressures of the gases in the cylinders vary from 700 to 2,000 lb./sq. in. Such pressures are, of course, not manageable when metering the gases through the anaesthetic machine and they must be reduced to workable levels. The Adams' Valve (Fig. 14) is commonly used for this purpose. Each valve bears colours similar to the cylinder for which it is intended and is also labelled with the name of the appropriate gas. It bears pins which will fit into the holes drilled in the head of the cylinder fitting only the corresponding cylinder.

The nitrous oxide and carbon dioxide valves in addition have fluting on them which presents a larger surface for absorption of heat since the nitrous oxide and carbon dioxide are changing from a liquid to a gas and therefore absorbing heat. Without the fluting the reducing valve might freeze and cease to function.

Flow Meters

The flow meters in common use are known as rotameters. They consist of tapered glass tubes in which spin aluminium bobbins (Fig. 15). The spinning bobbin is not in contact with the side of the tube and is therefore unlikely to stick. This avoids false readings of gas flow. The gas flow is indicated by the figure on the rotameter opposite the top of the bobbin.

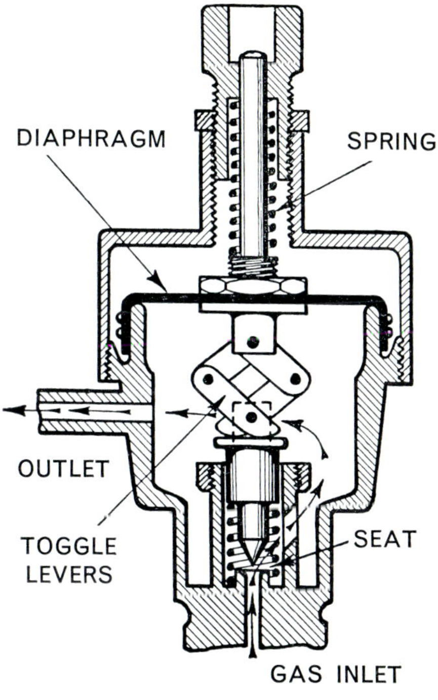

FIG. 14

Working principle of Adams' valve. When the outlet is occluded the pressure on the valve rises, the diaphragm lifts and the toggle levers force the pin into the valve seat stopping the flow of gas from the cylinder.

Vaporisers

These may be divided into two types. The simple vaporiser (Fig. 16) is suitable for vaporisation of trichloroethylene and ether where the exact concentration of the vapour emitted is not critical. A lever at the side of the bottle directs an increasing amount of the gas into the bottle and when the plunger is depressed the stream of gases coming up the J tube is directed on to or indeed through the fluid in the bottle.

Many factors govern the concentration of volatile anaesthetic given off from a simple vaporiser. Among these are:—

1. Ambient pressure and temperature.
2. Temperature and vapour pressure of the agent.
3. Rate of carrier gas flow through the vaporiser.
4. Area of the gas liquid interface.
5. Position and movement of the vaporiser.

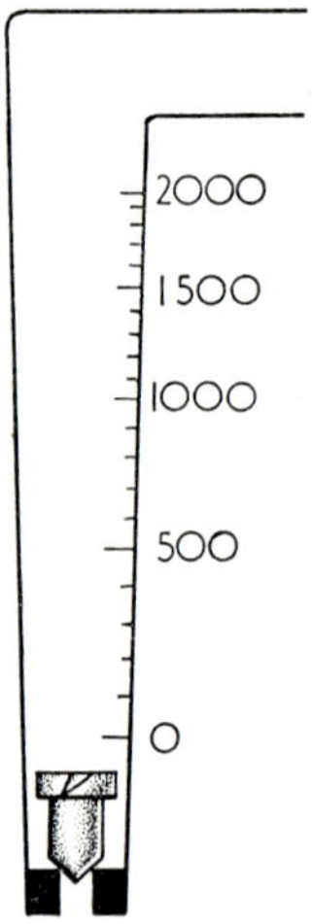

FIG. 15
The rotameter. As gas enters at the lower end the spinning bobbin rises in proportion to the flow of gas.

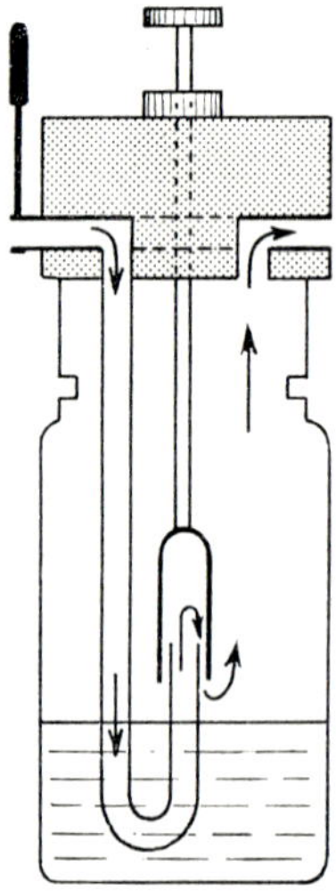

FIG. 16
A simple vaporiser—the Boyle's bottle. The arrows indicate the direction of gas flow.

The variations in these factors which may take place are quite considerable and are unacceptable when using a potent drug. The introduction of such potent anaesthetics and the increasing interest in using other anaesthetic agents in small, known concentrations has necessitated the use of more complicated vaporisers. One such vaporiser (Fig. 17) which automatically compensates for changes in the factors mentioned can deliver known concentrations of halothane in increments of 0·5 per cent. Similar vaporisers have been designed for use with chloroform, trichloroethylene, etc. The results using ether in a simple vaporiser and a compensated vaporiser are shown in Figure 18.

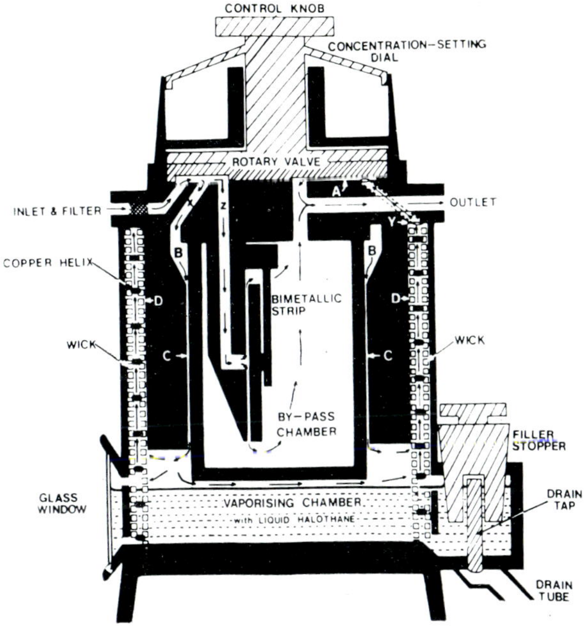

FIG. 17

The Fluotec Vaporiser Mark 3. This schematic diagram shows the construction of the vaporiser. The concentration-setting dial is in an 'ON' position. A=vapour control chamber; B=annular expansion chamber; C=long annular throat; D=spiral outlet channel of vaporising chamber; X=inlet to vaporising chamber; Y=outlet from vaporising chamber; Z=inlet to bypass chamber.

(From Paterson, G. M., Hulands, G. H. & Nunn, J. F. (1969). *British Journal of Anaesthesia* **41,** 109.)

Delivery of the Gases and Vapours to the Patient

This may be achieved by using a *Magill attachment* (Fig. 19) consisting of a corrugated rubber tube, a reservoir bag, and a spill valve. The reservoir is necessary since the flow of gas from the machine is continuous during all phases of respiration whereas the patient's demand for these gases is only during inspiration. At the patient's end of the tube is placed the uni-directional valve through which excess gas may pass and connection may be made with a mask which is placed over the patient's face.

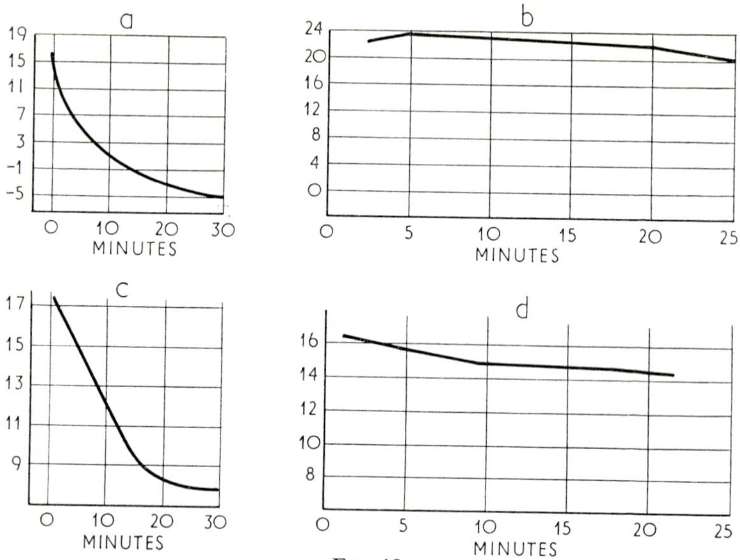

FIG. 18

The fall in temperature of liquid ether and decrease of ether vapour concentration in the output, when comparable gas flows are passed through a Boyle's bottle and a temperature compensated vaporiser.

(*a*) temperature change with time in Boyle's bottle (°C).
(*b*) minimal temperature change with time in a compensated vaporiser (°C).
(*c*) ether concentration change with time from a Boyle's bottle (vol. %).
(*d*) fairly constant ether concentration leaving a compensated vaporiser over a period of time (vol. %).

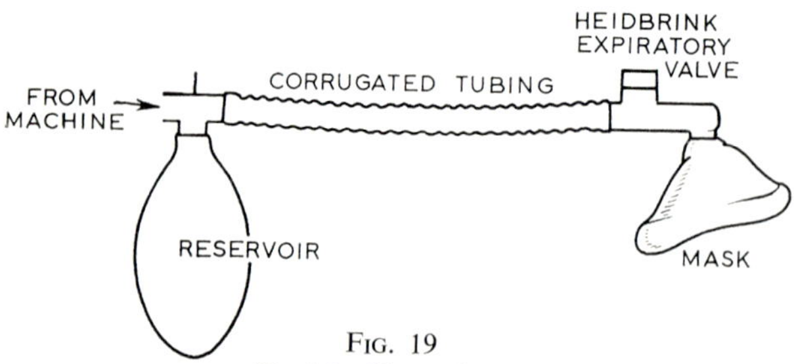

FIG. 19

The Magill attachment.

When using this type of circuit, it is necessary to deliver from the machine a flow of gases at least equal to the patient's minute volume (usually 8 litres/min.) otherwise carbon dioxide will accumulate and will be rebreathed. This system is best avoided when the patient's ventilation is being controlled.

A NON-RETURN OR NON-REBREATHING VALVE (Fig. 20) may be used instead of the conventional Heidbrink valve. In this case during expiration all the expired gas passes to the atmosphere and rebreathing of carbon dioxide is minimal.

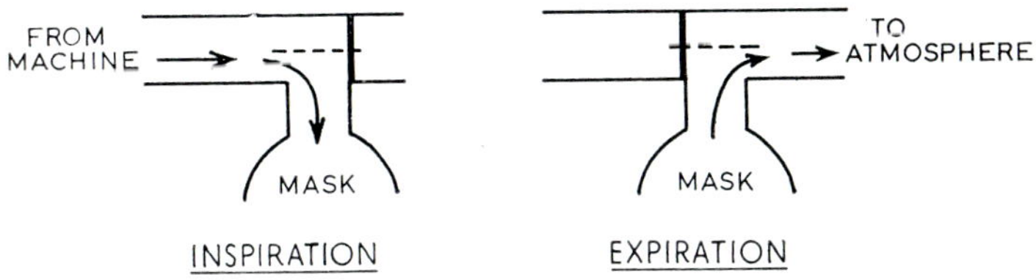

FIG. 20

A non-return valve. During inspiration the valve slides across and permits the patient to breathe gases from the machine. On expiration the valve cuts off the supply of gases from the machine and allows the expired gas from the patient to pass to the atmosphere.

THE T-PIECE CIRCUIT (Fig. 21) introduced by Ayre is used particularly in children where the resistance to expiration offered by valves is harmful to the child if spontaneous respiration takes place for a considerable time. The open limb of the T conveys expired gas to the atmosphere and acts as a reservoir.

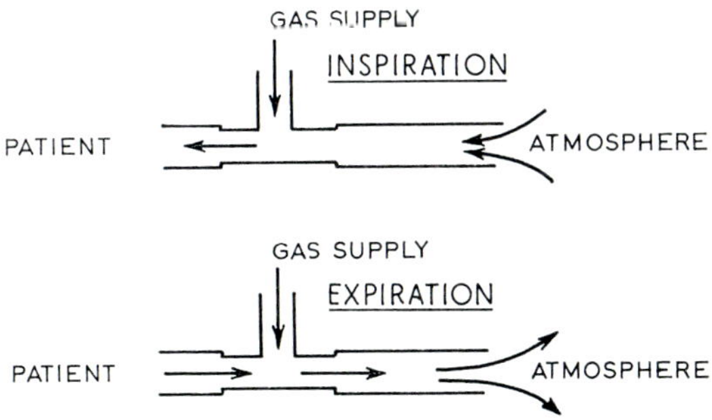

FIG. 21

The T-piece principle. As there are no valves, resistance is minimal and, by adjusting the flow of gases and the length of the expiratory limb to the atmosphere, the degree of rebreathing can be controlled.

A CLOSED CIRCUIT may also be used. Using such a system it is possible to pass the patient's expirate to the machine and back again, directing the expired gases through soda lime to absorb the carbon dioxide which is given off and adding oxygen as the gas is passed back to the patient (Fig. 22). Such a system offers several advantages.

1. Economy of gases and vapours.
2. Conservation of moisture and heat.
3. Avoidance of contamination of the theatre atmosphere with anaesthetic vapours.
4. Where inflammable agents are being used it minimises the risk of explosion.

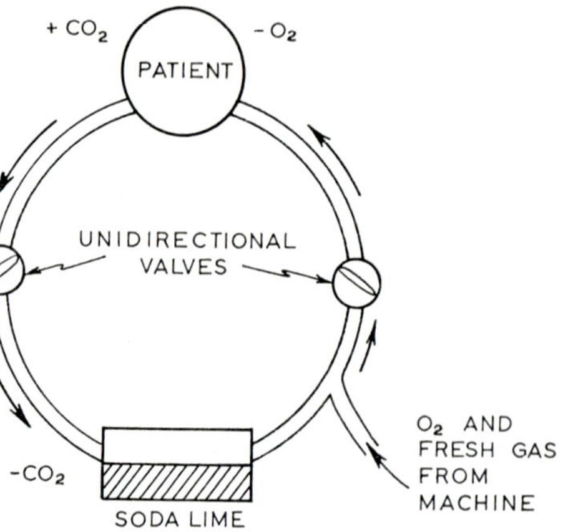

FIG. 22

Diagram of a closed circuit circle absorption system.

However, extra rubber tubing is required and valves must be interposed to keep the gases flowing in the correct direction. In addition the use of soda lime further increases the resistance to spontaneous respiration. During controlled ventilation this increase in resistance is less important. This system is not suitable for use with trichloroethylene which reacts with soda lime forming toxic products. It is also seldom used in children where the resistance is unacceptable.

Nowadays many anaesthetists use the " closed circuit " with a flow of gases higher than basal oxygen requirements. This means that a valve must be introduced into the circuit and some gases spilled to the outside air. This is less economical than a completely closed circuit but it does minimise the chance of a dangerous concentration of gas or vapour being built up and is said to be more efficient in ensuring the removal of carbon dioxide than reliance on the absorber alone.

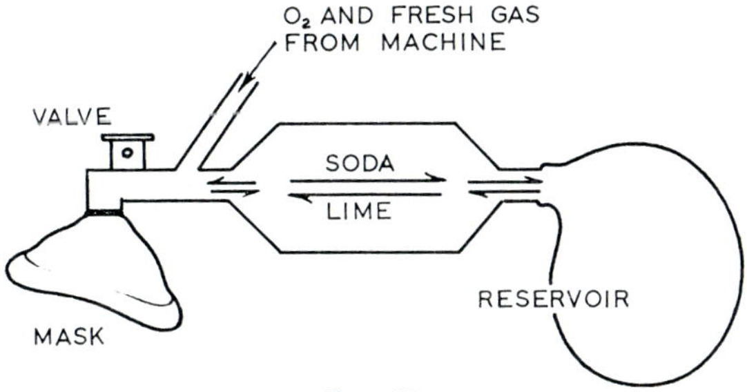

FIG. 23
The Waters anaesthetic circuit. The gases pass to and fro through the soda lime canister.

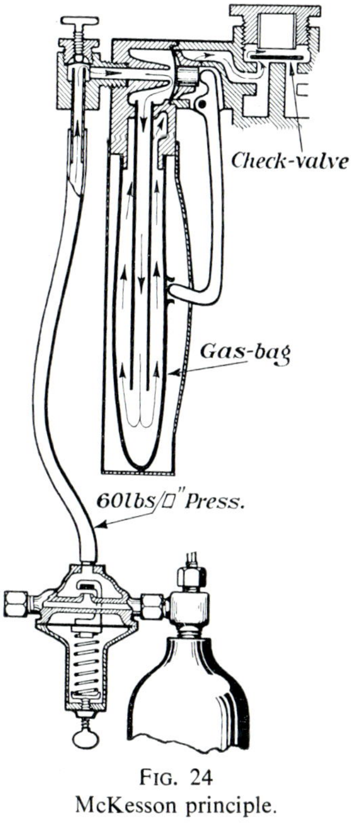

FIG. 24
McKesson principle.

In addition to the type of closed circuit system illustrated, it is possible to use a more portable system depending on the passage of gases to and fro through a Waters canister (Fig. 23). This system while more portable is more cumbersome to use and is declining in popularity in this country.

Intermittent Flow Machines

Most of the anaesthetic machines used in this country are based on the continuous flow principle—that is the gas flows at a constant rate throughout all phases of respiration, the excess during expiration being accommodated in a reservoir. Other machines, however, used for general purposes (e.g. the McKesson machine) for dental anaesthesia (e.g. the Walton machine) and for obstetric analgesia (e.g. the Minnitt machine) supply gases to the patient only during inspiration.

A check valve (Fig. 24) causes the supply of gases to be cut off when the pressure rises in the reservoir. It is essential when using such a machine to ensure that a gas-tight fit is obtained between the patient's face and the mask, or the machine will not function satisfactorily.

OTHER METHODS OF ADMINISTRATION

The Open Mask

The Schimmelbusch mask (Fig. 25), originally introduced for use with chloroform, consists of a base with a frame over which a layer of lint is normally placed. The shape of the frame does not allow a gas-tight fit and thus air or oxygen can be drawn in between the face and the mask. It could also be used to administer ether to small children.

Ether, however, can also be given on an Ogston mask (Fig. 26). Here several layers of gauze are put over the frame and a towel is pinned round the built-up portion to ensure that some vapour is retained above the gauze and reinhaled along with accumulated carbon dioxide to act as a respiratory stimulant. In addition a gas-tight fit is obtained by placing over the face a gamgee pad with a hole cut in it through which the patient breathes. This ensures that all inspiration and expiration takes place through the gauze.

Draw-over Vaporisers

While the methods described above had the great advantage of extreme portability, they had many other disadvantages. Many of these can be overcome by using a draw-over inhaler such as the Oxford vaporiser developed during the Second

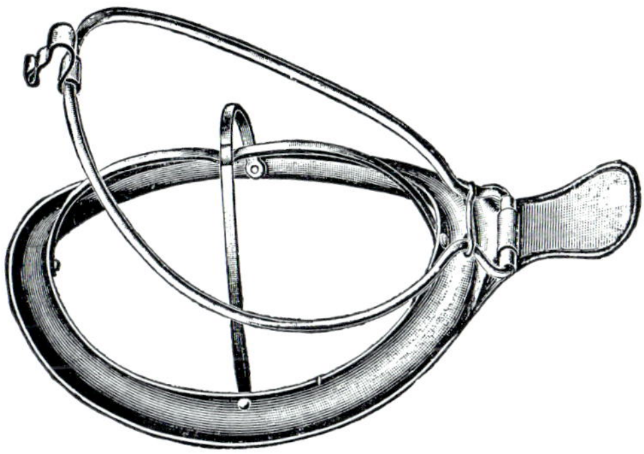

FIG. 25
Schimmelbusch's mask.

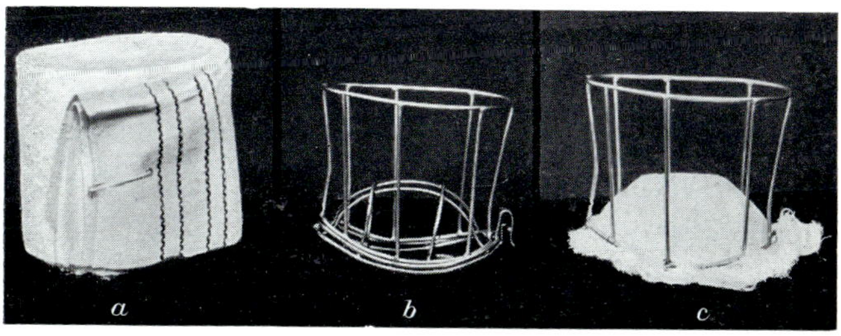

FIG. 26
Ogston's ether inhaler. (*a*) Inhaler fully draped and ready for use. (*b*) Frame of inhaler. (*c*) Inhaler with gauze only, but before towel is pinned round uprights.

World War. No cylinders are required and as the patient inhales, air is drawn from the atmosphere through the inhaler, vaporising the ether in carefully controlled concentrations. Other vaporisers which compensate for temperature changes have been developed also in Oxford and may be used where anaesthetic gases or special apparatus are unavailable. Such inhalers have been used for all types of surgery in all types of patients.

Trichloroethylene in air is used as an analgesic in obstretrics. Vaporisers compensated for temperature changes deliver small, known concentrations of trichloroethylene in air to the patient.

CHAPTER IV

PRE-ANAESTHETIC EXAMINATION AND THERAPY INCLUDING PREMEDICATION

Anaesthetic Outpatient Clinic

Ideally, all patients should be seen at an anaesthetic outpatient clinic at about the time that they are seen at the surgical outpatient clinic. This enables many conditions requiring treatment, such as anaemia, chronic bronchitis and dental sepsis to be detected by an anaesthetist before the patient is admitted, thus saving time and beds. In some hospitals all patients requiring surgery are referred to the anaesthetist while in others only patients whose condition seems likely to require pre-operative therapy are referred for this purpose. In other hospitals the anaesthetist may attend the surgical outpatient clinic.

Few hospitals have such facilities, however, and in most cases the examination and treatment of patients in the pre-anaesthetic period takes place after their admission to hospital for surgery.

Pre-anaesthetic Examination

The object of this examination is to detect any abnormality which will increase the risks of surgery and anaesthesia.

A. The Patient is Closely Questioned, special attention being paid to the following.

1. *The mode of life.* Note is taken here of the patient's occupation, his habits as regards exercise, alcohol and tobacco.

2. *Previous illnesses.* Of particular importance are those which may have left some damage, for example, rheumatic fever or diphtheria.

In addition, note is taken of any history of asthma or other allergic disease and other more unusual conditions such as porphyria.

3. *Drug therapy.* Details are sought of any drugs which the patient is taking or has been taking during the previous two years. Specially important are steroids, sedatives and drugs affecting the cardiovascular system, particularly hypotensive agents.

4. *Previous anaesthetic experiences.* Note any complications which have occurred and the personal preferences of each patient for individual techniques.

5. *The surgical condition for which the operation is proposed.* Elicit any symptoms or signs which may be relevant to the anaesthetic, for example a patient who has been bleeding copiously may well be anaemic when he comes to surgery.

6. *Symptoms suggestive of cardio-respiratory insufficiency or disease.* Leading questions are directed to symptoms such as cough, breathlessness on exertion, swelling of the ankles, etc.

While taking this history the anaesthetist has an opportunity to assess the patient's nervous temperament and this will give him some guide in prescribing pre-operative sedative medication.

B. SYSTEMATIC EXAMINATION OF THE PATIENT is then undertaken.

1. *The respiratory system.* While the patient's history regarding cough, breathlessness on exertion and his degree of exercise tolerance is of considerable importance in assessing his fitness for anaesthesia, routine clinical examination of the lungs is carried out. A case can be made out also for routine chest radiography in all patients undergoing major surgery. Where the history or examination indicates limitation of function or limitation of exercise tolerance, special respiratory function tests may be carried out. These are discussed separately (p. 63). If the patient has a cough a specimen of sputum should be obtained and examined for organisms and sensitivity to antibiotics.

2. *The cardiovascular system.* Here again the history is of considerable importance in assessing the state of the heart and circulation. A routine clinical examination is, however, carried out including measurement of the blood pressure and of the haemoglobin level. Where indicated electrocardiography and other special tests may also be carried out (p. 61).

3. *The urinary system.* The urine is examined chemically and microscopically for any abnormal constituents such as sugar, albumen, blood or cells. Where any of these are present further investigation of the urinary tract is undertaken. In

many cases, particularly those undergoing major surgery, the blood urea is estimated.

4. *Nutrition and hydration.* In most patients admitted for elective surgery, little abnormal will be noted in this respect but in patients who have been suffering from wasting diseases or who have been vomiting or losing fluids from fistulae it is important that blood should be sent for estimation of the plasma proteins, electrolytes, liver function tests and acid-base measurements.

5. *The system to be operated on* should be examined if this is likely to have a particular bearing on the anaesthetic.

6. *The nose, throat and teeth should be carefully examined* for signs of deformity or infection which may influence the maintenance of an airway. In addition, the superficial veins should be carefully examined if an intravenous induction of anaesthesia is planned. Where it is intended to use a regional analgesic technique, the area of the contemplated injection should be carefully studied lest there are contraindications to the use of such a technique.

Having examined the patient fully the overall picture of his physical status may be established. The American Society of Anesthesiology classify physical status in the pre operative period as follows:—

Class 1. A normal healthy patient.
Class 2. A patient with a mild systemic disease.
Class 3. A patient with a severe systemic disease that limits activity but is not incapacitating.
Class 4. A patient with an incapacitating systemic disease that is a constant threat to life.
Class 5. A moribund patient not expected to survive 24 hours with or without operation.

This method of grading the patient is often helpful in impressing on all concerned the necessity for energetic pre-operative treatment or occasionally for postponing operative treatment.

Preparation for Anaesthesia and Operation

A. TREATMENT OF ESTABLISHED LESIONS.

1. *Where the patient has an acute respiratory infection,* operation should be postponed where at all possible. The likelihood of post-operative chest complications is greatest

when an anaesthetic is given during the first three to four days of a common cold—the so-called invasive period. If the operation cannot be delayed an antibiotic may be given to reduce the danger of secondary bacterial invasion.

2. *Patients with a chronic respiratory condition* should, where possible, be operated on during a period of remission, normally in the spring and summer. Physiotherapy, in the form of breathing exercises, should be given pre-operatively and may usefully be combined with exhibition of broncho-dilator drugs. If the sputum is infected, appropriate chemotherapy should be given and, in severe cases, blood gas levels should be estimated to act as a base line for post-operative therapy.

3. *Where the patient is found to be anaemic,* it may be possible to institute iron therapy and re-admit him later when his haemoglobin has reached acceptable levels. If this is not possible then the patient may be given blood or preferably packed red cells, and a period of three days allowed to elapse before operation as it has been shown that transfused blood does not reach its maximum oxygen carrying capacity for this period. Elective surgery should seldom be undertaken where the haemoglobin level is below 70 per cent., Sahli (10-10·5 G.Hb./100 ml.). In this connection it is worth remembering that one bottle of blood normally raises the haemoglobin level by about 8 per cent., Sahli.

4. *The presence of uncomplicated hypertension* is not regarded as a serious contra-indication to a carefully given anaesthetic. In selected cases, rest in bed and sedation, normally with barbiturates, may be tried for a few days before operation.

5. *Cardiac decompensation* will necessitate active treatment with digitalis, diuretics, or other appropriate measures.

6. *Diabetics.* Patients who are under treatment with long acting insulins or with oral agents should be brought under control with soluble insulin on the day before operation. On the day of operation itself a glucose infusion is set up. *Never* give *oral* glucose pre-operatively. The urine is tested and insulin is given on the following sliding scale.

If the urine is blue, no insulin is given.

If the urine is green, ten units of soluble insulin are given subcutaneously.

If the urine is yellow, 20 units of soluble insulin are given.
If the urine is orange, 30 units of soluble insulin are given.

Post-operatively this regime is continued, the urine being tested three hourly, and only when the patient is stabilised on diet are long acting agents restarted.

7. *Patients who have been on prolonged steroid therapy* should be considered as special anaesthetic risks. Anaesthesia, surgery and post-operative complications are considerable stresses for which the patient may be unable to compensate and this must be allowed for when prescribing supplementary steroid therapy. Even if steroid therapy has been discontinued for some time prior to surgery the patient may still be at risk. The extent to which a patient is able to respond to stress may be determined by measuring plasma cortisol levels before and after an injection of A.C.T.H.

8. *Many patients are on some form of sedative therapy.* These drugs may affect the course of anaesthesia in one of two ways. Patients who are receiving phenothiazine derivatives such as chlorpromazine may require very little thiopentone and, indeed, if more than minimal doses of this drug are given, marked hypotension and prolonged recovery may follow. On the other hand, patients who are habituated to barbiturates or to alcohol may be very resistant to normal doses of anaesthetic agents and induction may prove difficult in such cases. Recently a further hazard has been revealed. Diazepam has been shown to increase the intensity and duration of the neuromuscular block produced by non-depolarising drugs.

The monoamine oxidase inhibitor group of drugs used in the treatment of depression may cause:—

(*a*) Severe hypertension, particularly after amphetamine-like drugs.

(*b*) Abnormal reactions—hypotension, hypertension and hyperpyrexia—to narcotics.

(*c*) Delayed recovery of consciousness after general anaesthesia.

(*d*) Liver damage.

These drugs listed below should be stopped for as long as possible before anaesthesia.

Approved name	*Proprietary name*
Isocarboxazid	Marplan
Mebanazine	Actomol
Pheniprazine	Cavodil
Phenoxypropazine	Drazine
Pargyline*	Eutonyl
Iproniazid	Marsilid
Phenelzine	Nardil
Nialamide	Niamid
Tranylcypromine*	Parnate
Tranylcypromine* and Trifluoperazine	Parstelin
Pivhydrazine	Tersavid

Most of these drugs are hydrazine derivatives; the two exceptions are marked with an asterisk *.

9. *Hypotensive Agents.* Patients on hypotensive therapy present a problem to the anaesthetist. If such a patient is anaesthetised, profound falls in blood pressure which may not respond to vasopressor therapy may be encountered. If, on the other hand, hypotensive therapy is discontinued the patient is submitted to surgery with an increased strain on his myocardium, a reduced blood volume, and the risks from these states are added to the operative risk.

Hypotensive drugs differ in their site of action and the duration of action after withdrawal. The duration of action of some of the commoner drugs is as follows:—

Pargyline (Eutonyl)	14 days
Methoserpidine (Decaserpyl)	14 days
Guanethidine (Ismelin)	10-12 days
Methyldopa (Aldomet)	7-10 days
Veratrum (Veriloid)	7 days
Pempidine (Perolysen) (Tenormal)	4 days
Guanoxan (Envacar)	4 days
Bethanidine (Esbatal)	1 day
Guanoclor (Vatensol)	1 day
Mecamylamine (Inversine) (Mevasine)	1 day

In the presence of renal damage these periods of action should be doubled.

Many of the patients who are on hypotensive therapy may also be receiving diuretics and this may result in potassium depletion with alteration in the response to muscle relaxant drugs.

It is important to discover that a patient is receiving hypotensive drugs early, at his out-patient visit if possible. In the mild hypertensive, long-acting drugs may be discontinued and replaced by mild sedation and bed rest. In more severe cases the longer-acting drug is replaced by a hypotensive drug of shorter action, e.g. bethanidine.

10. *Antibiotics* in large doses may potentiate the curariform drugs. All " mycin " drugs, e.g. neomycin and streptomycin, are particularly important in this respect.

11. *Oral contraceptives* may inhibit the breakdown of pethidine in the body and should clearly be stopped pre-operatively.

12. *Where examination reveals alteration in the plasma proteins* or unsatisfactory electrolyte levels, intravenous therapy should be commenced to ensure that these deficiencies are remedied before anaesthesia and operation.

The treatment of the lesions detailed above may be started a few days before anaesthesia is contemplated and we may now pass to the more immediate preparation of the patient.

Written permission for anaesthesia must always be obtained. In Britain an individual of 16 years of age or over may give consent for treatment without the authority of a parent or guardian, provided he is capable of understanding what this treatment involves. The consent of a parent or guardian should however be obtained where the patient is under the age of 16. In an emergency every reasonable effort should be made to obtain written consent but where the patient is, for example, unconscious or relatives are not readily available, essential treatment should not be withheld.

Consent to anaesthesia and operation should be informed—i.e. the purpose of the operation should be explained to the patient or parent. Whenever possible the consent form should be kept in the patient's record folder and be checked by the anaesthetist.

B. ROUTINE PREPARATION.

1. *It is essential to ensure that every patient goes to theatre with an empty stomach.* Of the small number of deaths each

year which may be attributed to anaesthesia, one in every eight is due to the patient vomiting or regurgitating during anaesthesia. All these deaths must be regarded as preventable. Normally, no food or fluid is given to the patient by mouth for a period of at least four hours pre-operatively. In addition, it is essential to ensure that the patient knows why this is being done and to see that he does not eat or drink from stores in his locker. In the case of children, who cannot be relied upon to obey these instructions, food and fluid should be removed from their lockers in the pre-operative period.

In some cases this period of fasting may be impossible or may be considered to be unsatisfactory. This is so

(*a*) when operation is contemplated shortly after a meal has been ingested,

(*b*) in certain conditions where it is known that the stomach fills up from below as, for instance, in intestinal obstruction, or

(*c*) under certain circumstances in which it is known that the emptying of the stomach is delayed.

Although more than four hours may have elapsed since the patient has last taken food or fluid by mouth, the stomach may still contain food ingested many hours before, if an injury has been sustained shortly after the meal, i.e. before the stomach has emptied. Under these circumstances it is essential that active steps are taken to empty the stomach. Normally, where food has been taken a large bore stomach tube is passed and, where the alimentary tract is intact, lavage using saline may be used to assist in emptying the stomach. Where food has not been taken but the stomach is considered to contain fluid, an oesophageal tube may be employed instead of the stomach tube. Under no circumstances should a Ryle's tube be employed. This tube is intended only to remove gastric juice for testing and is of too narrow a bore to empty a full stomach.

The oral administration of an antacid to neutralise gastric acidity is often of value even where the stomach is thought to be virtually empty. Even a small quantity of acid, if regurgitated and inhaled, may jeopardise the patient's life (see p. 130).

An alternative method of emptying the stomach is to induce vomiting by giving apomorphine intravenously. In this way solid food can be more easily recovered from the stomach. The method is, however, unpleasant and in patients who are very ill may be dangerous. Profuse salivation and bradycardia accompany the vomiting, which may be prolonged, and intravenous atropine may be required to antagonise these effects. In very few centres is apomorphine used as an alternative to the mechanical methods of emptying the stomach.

2. *The bladder and bowel should be emptied* by the most appropriate means. Where major bowel surgery is contemplated enemata may have been given and where gynaecological or urological surgery is to be undertaken a catheter will have been passed before operation. It is, however, also essential to see that the outpatient, having even a light anaesthetic for a minor operation, is given the opportunity to empty his bladder and bowel lest he soil himself during the operation. Both the excitement associated with the operation and the anaesthetic agents employed may lead to emptying of the bladder during anaesthesia.

3. *Remove artificial teeth, contact lenses, rings, hairpins* and any other objects liable to harm the patient and also a watch which may be damaged during the operation.

4. *Administer the appropriate premedication.*

PREMEDICATION OR PRE-ANAESTHETIC MEDICATION

Premedication may be given for three reasons.

1. To relieve anxiety. This may include pain relief.
2. To abolish or reduce undesirable parasympathetic activity.
3. To reduce post-operative vomiting.

1. THE RELIEF OF ANXIETY OR SEDATION is nowadays the most important function of premedication. In some cases where pain is present pre-operatively, anxiety may be relieved by alleviating the pain. In other cases psychic sedation is what is aimed at.

Some time spent in reassurance and giving of simple explanations to the patient can save much in the way of drugs. Many patients will benefit from a simple explanation of hospital routine. They will appreciate being told that on the night before operation they will receive a hypnotic. They will also appreciate being told that, before going to theatre, pre-anaesthetic sedatives will be given so that they will approach the anaesthetic room with minimal anxiety. Many who have had previous surgery and have unpleasant memories of an inhalation induction will appreciate the promise of an intravenous induction. Despite the advent of medical television programmes, many patients know little of the routine of a surgical ward or theatre and their greatest fear is of the unknown.

While this psychological preparation is helpful, it is seldom in itself adequate to relieve anxiety and some form of sedative drug is normally given.

In very nervous patients, a mild sedative may be given for a few days before admission and certainly soon after admission rather than allowing uncontrolled anxiety to persist until one hour pre-operatively.

The choice of sedative used in the immediate pre-operative period is largely determined by the aims of the anaesthetist. The opiates are still widely used because, particularly combined with hyoscine, they relieve anxiety and also provide some analgesia in the immediate post-operative period. A wide variety of non-analgesic sedatives is in use and these may be combined with a small dose of analgesic (see p. 26).

Sedation is further discussed on page 163.

2. PARASYMPATHETIC OVERACTIVITY during anaesthesia may manifest itself as bradycardia, excessive secretion of saliva and bronchial mucus or as broncho-constriction. Although, with the use of modern agents, irritation of the bronchi with excessive secretion is less common, and the routine use of a belladonna derivative is now being questioned, many anaesthetists still include such a drug in their premedication. The drugs commonly used are atropine sulphate or hyoscine hydrobromide (Scopolamine).

Atropine in appropriate dosage may be given to patients of all ages but has no sedative properties. *Hyoscine* on the other hand provides a welcome amnesia, the patients remembering little of what has happened to them. Its disadvantages are that it has no vagolytic action and indeed may cause slight cardiac slowing. In older patients it may cause restlessness and confusion and its use is usually restricted to patients under the age of 60.

Often, the atropine or hyoscine is incorporated in the premedication given about one hour pre-operatively. However, some anaesthetists, to avoid giving the patient a dry mouth during this period, omit the belladonna derivative from the original injection and instead inject it intravenously at the time of induction.

More detailed pharmacology of many of these drugs was discussed at page 26.

3. POST-OPERATIVE VOMITING arises for many reasons but some reduction in its incidence may be obtained by the use of appropriate drugs in premedication. Such a drug is hyoscine and this agent has been used widely in preventing motion sickness. Alternatively, the phenothiazines, cyclizine, droperidol or metoclopramide, may be given in an attempt to reduce the incidence of post-operative vomiting. They may be given alone or in combination with other drugs. Some anaesthetists give a small dose of promethazine several hours before the main premedication.

Timing and Administration of Premedication

The opiates and atropine are non-irritant solutions and may be given subcutaneously about one to one and a half hours pre-operatively. Many of the other drugs used, such as pethidine and the phenothiazines, are more irritant and are normally given by intramuscular injection thirty to forty minutes pre-operatively. This route should also be used where the patient is obese or if inadequate time is available to give the drug subcutaneously. It is useless and indeed positively dangerous to give premedication at a time when it cannot possibly be absorbed before the induction of anaesthesia. Not only does the patient gain no benefit from the sedatives incorporated in it but these drugs will exert their maximum depressant activity during anaesthesia when depression from other agents is already maximal. If for any reason the injections have not been given at the prescribed time intervals, the drugs should be withheld and given intravenously by the anaesthetist. Normally, the sedative is omitted at this stage and only a belladonna derivative is given.

ORAL PREMEDICATION is at first sight a contradiction of the normal routine that nothing is given to a patient by mouth in the four hours preceding surgery. The obvious attraction, however, of avoiding injections particularly in children has led to a revival of the practice of giving premedication by mouth. Apart from the disadvantage of having to swallow a tablet, capsule or syrup with the accompanying fluid required, in a patient starved of fluid and anxious, absorption from the stomach is variable. The drugs used are usually trimeprazine (Vallergan), barbiturates, non-barbiturate hypnotics or the tranquillisers such as chlordiazepoxide. All are non-analgesic preparations but are effective over a period of up to four hours so that the timing of oral premedication is not so critical.

Identification of Patients

It is vitally important that all patients going to theatre should bear adequate means of identification. This is becoming ever more important in view of the increasing work load falling on units which may be short staffed. The possibility of operating on the wrong patient or carrying out the wrong operation is increased under these circumstances. Identification is usually accomplished by attaching to the patient's wrist a label which bears his name, age and address. Ideally this label should be attached to the patient soon after his admission to hospital. Care must also be taken to ensure that all concerned know what operation is proposed and, where an operation may be performed on either side such as ligation of varicose veins or herniorrhaphy, it is clearly understood which side is to be operated on. It is, therefore, wise to check with each patient immediately before the induction of anaesthesia which side has been causing him trouble.

CHAPTER V

SPECIAL PRE-OPERATIVE INVESTIGATIONS

While this subject can be conveniently considered in two parts, i.e. the assessment of cardiac function and the assessment of pulmonary function, such a division is artificial since the two are closely related and can never be properly considered in isolation.

ASSESSMENT OF CARDIAC FUNCTION

The practice of labelling patients as " cardiac " and managing each case in a routine fashion is to be condemned. The type of cardiac disease, the functional capacity of the heart and the presence or absence of decompensation, i.e. cardiac failure, are the three factors of importance in the assessment and anaesthetic management of the patient. These patients should be regarded as suffering primarily from cardiac disease with a complicating surgical disease rather than the reverse.

The great bulk of so-called " cardiacs " who come before the anaesthetist are suffering from degenerative cardio-vascular disease. In the absence of recent decompensation, myocardial infarction or accompanying renal disease, they present few problems to the anaesthetist, provided care is taken to avoid hypoxic techniques and drugs known to cause myocardial depression. In addition, there is increasing evidence that elderly patients, with degenerative cardiovascular disease but no frank cardiac failure, may benefit from pre-operative digitalisation.

Valvular disease, in the absence of cardiac failure, is not a contra-indication to surgery and anaesthesia. Congenital cardiac disease is uncommonly associated with failure and with reasonable care these patients give little trouble.

What methods can we use to assess the patient's fitness for operation? There is no substitute for the complete and careful clinical examination of the patient combined with accurate history taking. This is supplemented by various *standard investigations,* e.g. electrocardiography: X-ray: simple exercise

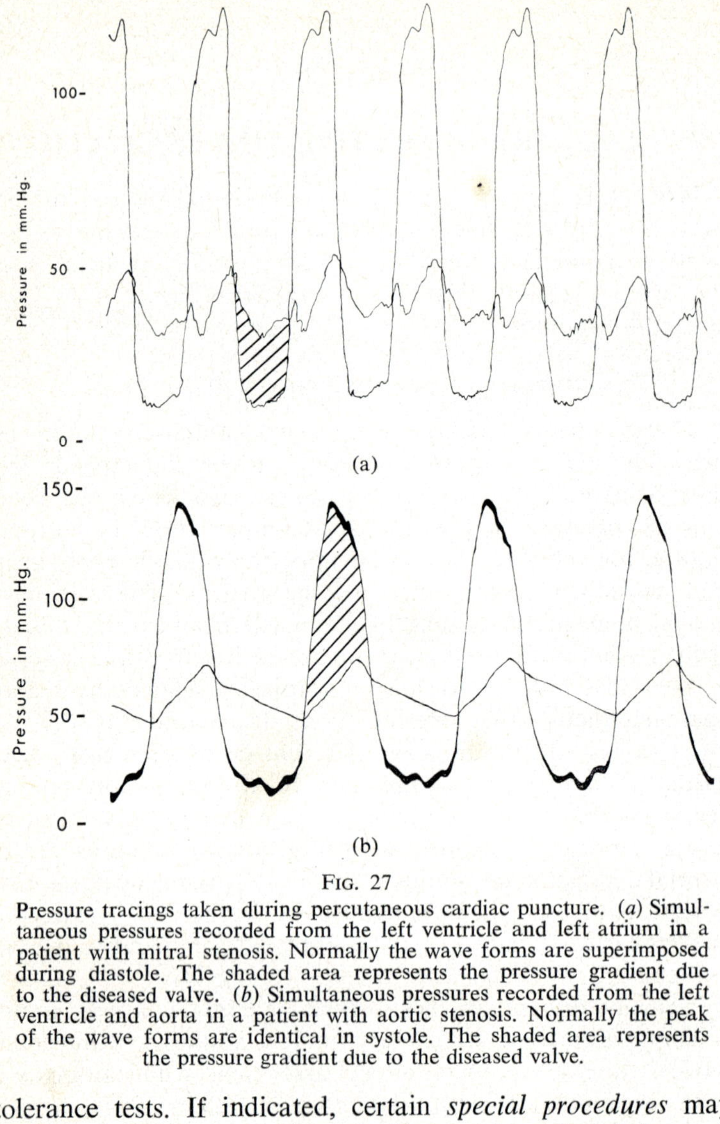

FIG. 27

Pressure tracings taken during percutaneous cardiac puncture. (*a*) Simultaneous pressures recorded from the left ventricle and left atrium in a patient with mitral stenosis. Normally the wave forms are superimposed during diastole. The shaded area represents the pressure gradient due to the diseased valve. (*b*) Simultaneous pressures recorded from the left ventricle and aorta in a patient with aortic stenosis. Normally the peak of the wave forms are identical in systole. The shaded area represents the pressure gradient due to the diseased valve.

tolerance tests. If indicated, certain *special procedures* may be used, e.g. cardiac catheterisation, angiocardiography, oximetry before and after exercise and measurement of cardiac output by dye dilution tests. In some cases further information may be required to elucidate the condition. This is particularly true where valvular disease is known to exist and where surgical correction of this disease is contemplated. Accurate information about the pressures in various chambers of the heart and the degree of valvular stenosis or incompetence can be obtained by the technique of cardiac puncture (Fig. 27). This investigation may be combined with estimation of cardiac output by sampling blood from the various parts of the heart and by measuring the oxygen consumption by spirometry.

It will be seen that with the above approach to the assessment of these cases, a very complete picture of each patient's fitness for any surgical procedure can be readily obtained. Unfortunately, until recently this logical approach has not been used by clinicians when faced with the problem of assessing the lung function of surgical patients.

ASSESSMENT OF LUNG FUNCTION

Professor Melville-Arnott said, " Clinicians seem curiously reluctant to use physiological lines of thought in the analysis and treatment of respiratory diseases. The current clinical approach is still dominated by ' stony dullness ' and ' dry sounds '." That this is wrong and unnecessary is evident when one considers that for many years now physiologists have used fairly simple techniques of assessing lung function. It is becoming increasingly obvious that it is essential for the physician, surgeon and anaesthetist to understand the functional changes in the lungs and their significance from the point of view of diagnosis, therapy and surgery.

Almost every technique the anaesthetist employs and almost every drug administered has some effect on respiration. For example, the widely employed method of intermittent positive pressure ventilation or " controlled " ventilation would be hazardous in the extreme and certainly not controlled if the anaesthetist were ignorant of the basic oxygen requirements of his patient and the need to ensure elimination of the end product of respiration, carbon dioxide. Again, morphine is a drug commonly used for premedication. The anaesthetist must be aware that this drug is a powerful respiratory depressant throughout the therapeutic dose range, raising the respiratory threshold to carbon dioxide stimulation. This effect may seriously interfere with a patient's ability to compensate for changes in metabolism by increasing alveolar ventilation.

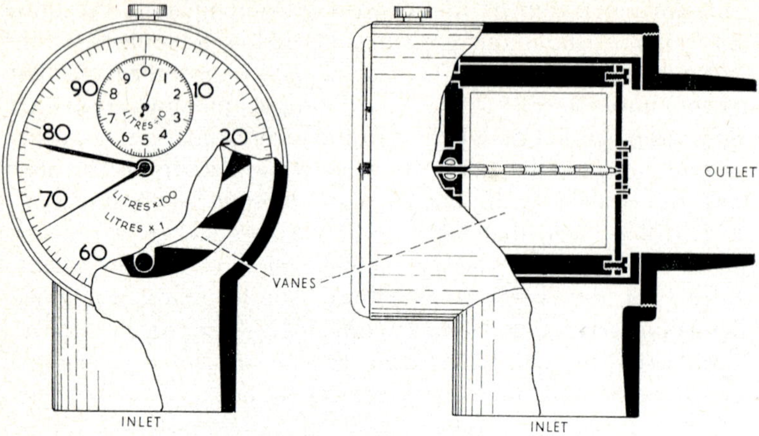

FIG. 28A
This diagram shows the working principle of the Wright respirometer. Gases passing via the inlet, drive the vanes and the flow is recorded on the dials.

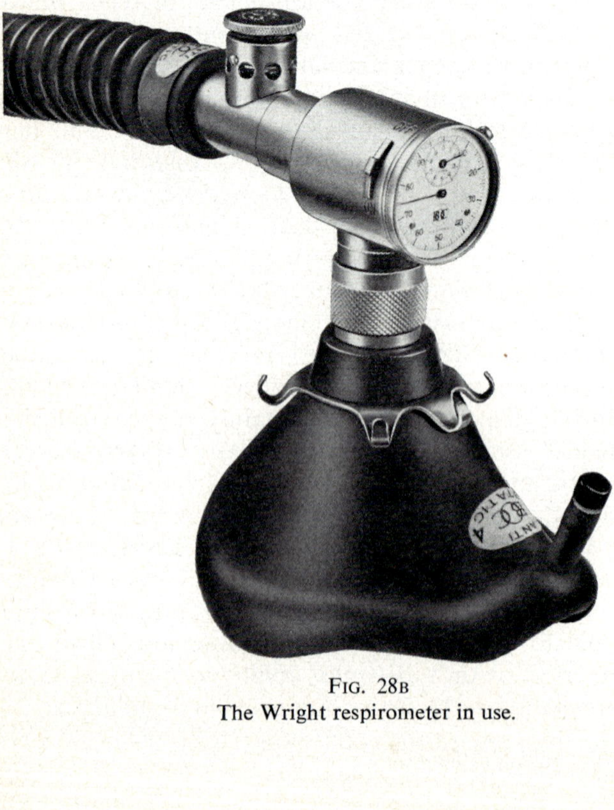

FIG. 28B
The Wright respirometer in use.

Lung function tests supplement the information obtained from the case history, examination and chest X-ray. Fortunately, the simplest of these tests measure exactly what the patient complains of most, that is inadequate *ventilatory function.* Impaired ventilation produces dyspnoea and is therefore much more noticeable than defects of the other three

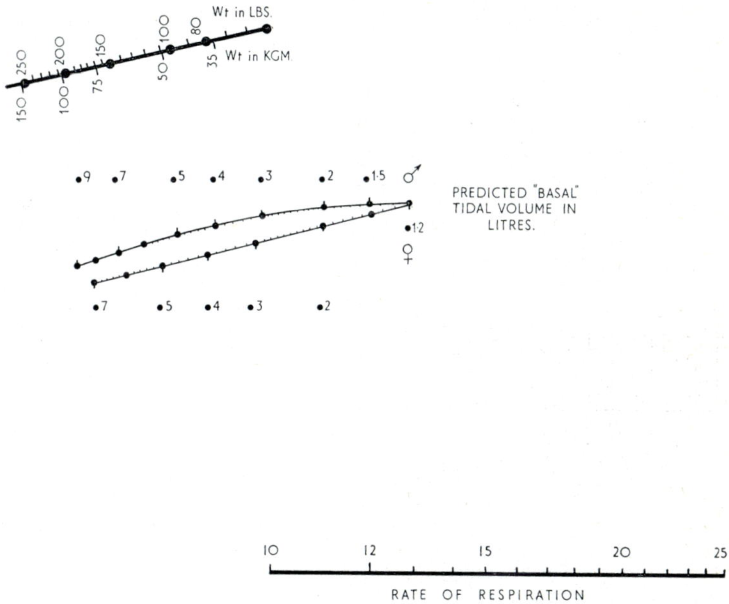

FIG. 29

The Radford Nomogram. A line drawn from the point, on the upper scale, indicating the patient's weight, to a point on the lower scale, representing the respiratory rate observed or desired, indicates the basal tidal volume where it bisects the middle lines.

divisions of lung function. The other three divisions are (1) *distribution of gases* in the lungs, (2) *exchange or diffusion of gases* across the alveolar capillary membrane, (3) the *pulmonary circulation* itself. Some of the tests for these three groups are at present complex but it is hoped to simplify them for use by the clinician.

The following are some tests in current clinical use.

Tidal Volume and Minute Volume

These can be measured now at the bedside by use of simple spirometers of the Drager or Wright type (Fig. 28) and yield useful information. The result can be compared with the expected normal predicted from tables or a nomogram (Fig. 29).

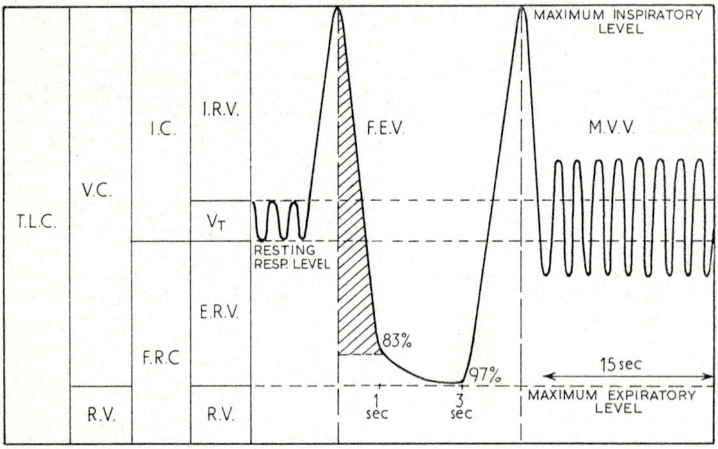

FIG. 30

This diagram or spirogram demonstrates the relationship of the various static lung volumes to the dynamic tests of lung function described in the text.

Symbol		*Normal Value in Adult Male*
V_T	= Tidal volume	500 mls.
I.C.	= Inspiratory capacity	3,600 mls.
E.R.V.	= Expiratory reserve volume	1,200 mls.
V.C.	= Vital capacity	4,800 mls.
R.V.	= Residual volume	1,200 mls.
F.R.C.	= Functional residual capacity	2,400 mls.
T.L.C.	= Total lung capacity	6,000 mls.

The following tests however are carried out by spirometry using an instrument which gives the clinician a permanent record of the patient's performance (Fig. 30).

Vital Capacity

This can be estimated in one or two stages, that is, inspiratory capacity plus expiratory reserve volume. Normal values can be calculated from a nomogram or a table giving average values for various age groups. The test is considered abnormal if the result is + or − 20 per cent. of the predicted value. Repeated tests are always done with the patient in the same posture. Normal values:—Male 4·78 litres, Female 3·14 litres. Reduction in vital capacity may not always be due to pulmonary disease, e.g. it may be due to (1) limitation of chest expansion, (2) limitation of descent of diaphragm, (3) limitation of expansion of lungs by effusions, etc. The test is of limited value as it is not dynamic, and the next test is an improvement.

Timed Vital Capacity

Alterations in the pattern of breathing become more apparent when maximal forced inspiratory and expiratory efforts are made. This is a simple test of *expiratory volume flow rate,* that is, it reflects the patient's ability to empty his lungs in a given time. The patient makes a forced expiration into a spirometer and this is timed. The volume in one, two or three seconds, can be expressed either as a percentage of tidal volume or as a percentage of predicted vital capacity. Normal values:—83 per cent. expired in one second, 94 per cent. in two seconds, 97 per cent. in three seconds.

The *Forced Expiratory Volume* or F.E.V. is that volume of gas expired between two stated time intervals (0-0·75 seconds) during the performance of the timed vital capacity.

Maximum Ventilatory Volume or Maximum Breathing Capacity

This is the maximum volume of gas in litres that can be breathed in one minute. As a general rule maximum ventilation can only be obtained by voluntary effort. The patient is instructed to breathe as deeply and as quickly as possible or as deeply as possible at a controlled rate. The test is usually done over 15 seconds since it is exhausting for a disabled patient. When neither rate nor depth are controlled, the test is referred to as free and the rate selected by the patient is noted. The M.V.V. can be calculated indirectly from the $F.E.V._{0.75}$ by multiplying by a factor of 40. Normal values:—Male aged 16 to 69 years 82-139 litres per minute; Female aged 16 to 69 years 63·6-101·5 litres per minute. The test is difficult, and the M.V.V. is usually calculated indirectly from a single breath F.E.V.

Significance of These Tests

The ability of the patient to breathe at sustained high velocity depends on many factors, e.g. muscular force available, the stiffness of the lungs and thorax and the airway and tissue resistance. These tests are therefore not specific but provide a good deal of useful information for the clinician.

Peak Flow

The peak flow is the highest flow rate achieved by the patient during a forced expiration. This test is related to the F.E.V. and M.V.V. but the exact relationship is unimportant. The peak flow rate is a stable and reproducible measurement in its own right. The instrument used is illustrated (Fig. 31). One single forced expiration is all that is required and thus it is less tiring than M.V.V. to perform. The normal values for adults range from 500 ml. to 1,000 ml.

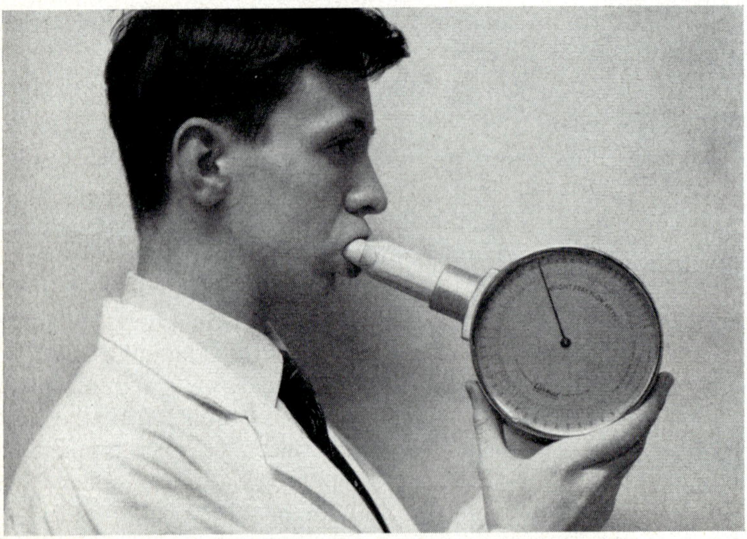

FIG. 31
The peak flow meter in use.

Blood Gas Analysis and Acid-Base Balance

Inadequate ventilation is reflected in changes in the oxygen content of the arterial blood and in alterations in the acid-base balance. The percentage saturation of the haemoglobin

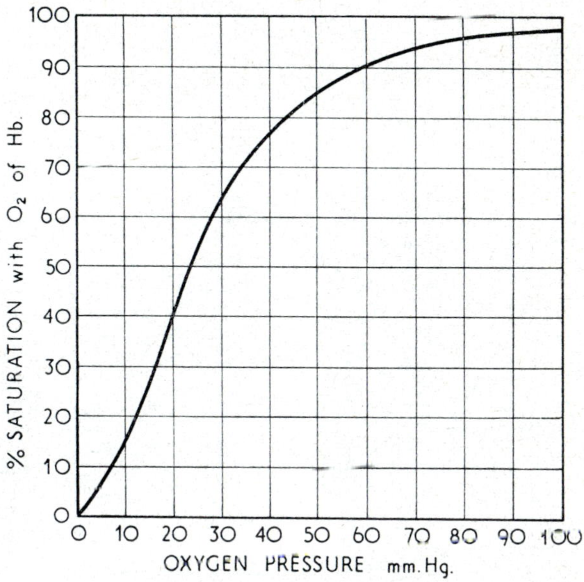

FIG. 32
The oxyhaemoglobin dissociation curve.

can be measured by the Van Slyke method. However, this method is cumbersome and slow and clinically the Haemo-reflector technique is now used. The measurement of the oxygen saturation of the arterial blood (Sa_{O_2}) is important in cases where inadequate ventilation is suspected since the clinical sign of cyanosis is not present until the oxygen saturation has fallen to about 70 per cent., the normal value being over 95 per cent.

On examination of the dissociation curve for haemoglobin (Fig. 32) it can be seen that hypoxia can exist even in the presence of what appears, at first sight, to be adequately oxygenated haemoglobin, e.g. an oxygen saturation of 90 per cent. corresponds to an arterial oxygen tension (Pa_{O_2}) of only 60 mm. Hg. It is a good practice to measure the P_{O_2} of the arterial blood in addition to the oxygen saturation. This can now be done with new electrodes that have been developed. The normal range of Pa_{O_2}, in a fit young adult, is 95-100 mm. Hg.

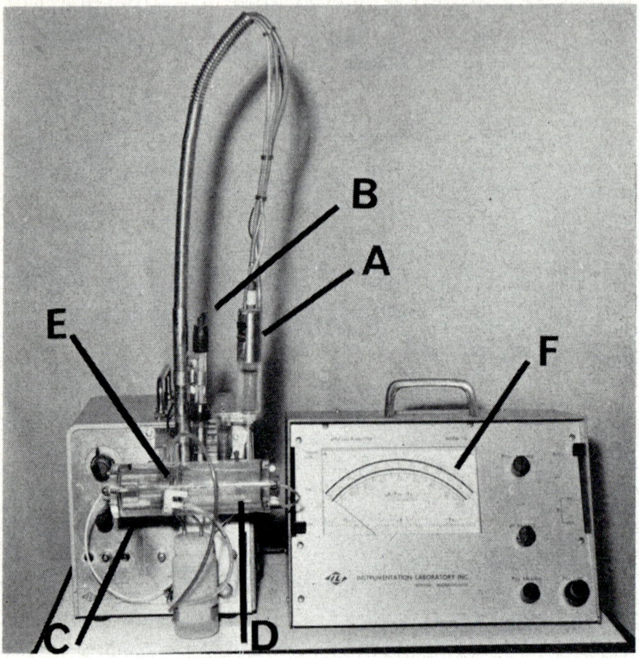

FIG. 33

The Instrumentation Laboratory Blood Gas Apparatus. A=pH measuring electrode with combined suction system. B=pH reference electrode; C=Po_2 electrode; D=Pco_2 electrode; E=cuvette for arterial blood sample; F=meter.

Until recently it was difficult and not clinically practicable to measure the changes in carbon dioxide tension (Pa_{CO_2}) and pH which follow upsets in pulmonary ventilation. A technique of measuring blood gas levels has now been developed which requires only a sample of capillary blood (Fig. 33).

There is a well recognised distinction between the two kinds of disturbance in the acid-base metabolism, the respiratory and the non-respiratory. Furthermore it is accepted that the P_{CO_2} of the arterial blood is the best measure of the respiratory disturbance as this tension is supposed to correspond with that of the alveolar air. The difficulty arises when we wish to choose an appropriate measure which will characterise the non-respiratory or metabolic disturbance only and which is uninfluenced by the changes in the acid base content of the blood caused by gross changes in pulmonary ventilation, i.e.

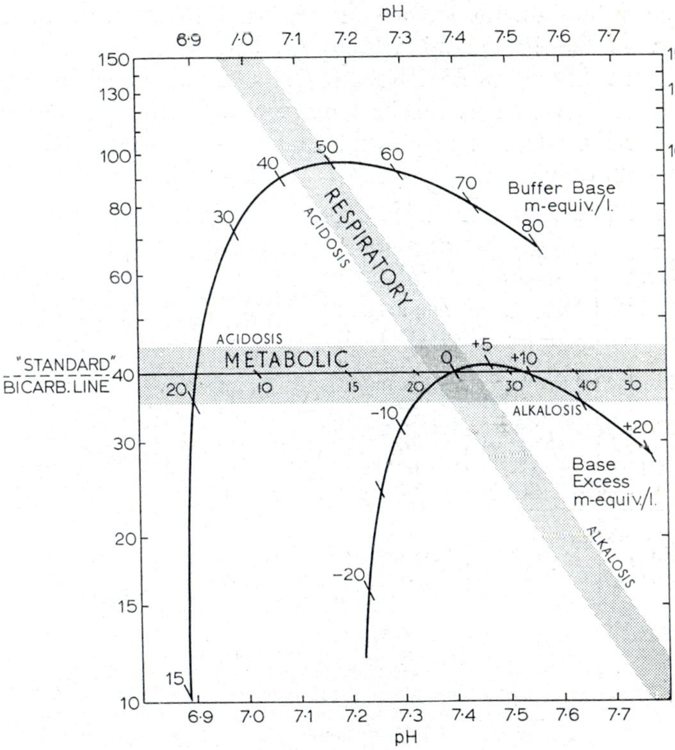

FIG. 34

The acid-base nomogram (after Siggaard Andersen). The shaded diagonal represents the respiratory component of the acid-base relationship, changes in an upward direction showing acidosis and in a downward direction alkalosis. The shaded horizontal line represents the metabolic component, acid changes being to the left and alkalotic to the right.

hypo- or hyper-ventilation. Many different measures have been employed in the past resulting in great confusion amongst clinicians and in an inability to compare results from one hospital to another and indeed between units in the same hospital, e.g. alkali reserve, total carbon dioxide of the plasma, carbon dioxide-combining power of the plasma and more recently the *Standard Bicarbonate*. This latter value is defined by Astrup as the " bicarbonate of true plasma separated from the blood with the haemoglobin completely oxygenated at a Pa_{CO_2} of 40 mm. Hg. and at body temperature (38° C.)." All the values mentioned above will vary in a given blood sample as the Pa_{CO_2} and arterial O_2 saturation are varied, except the Standard Bicarbonate. It is for this reason that it has been selected as the best measure when one wishes to eliminate the effect of respiration and measure the metabolic component only.

State	*pH (Units)*	*Respiratory Component* Pco_2 mm.Hg.	*Metabolic Component*	
			Standard bicarbonate m.Eq./litre	Base excess m.Eq./litre
Acidosis	Less than 7·36	More than 44	Less than 22	More than −2·5
Normal	7·36 to 7·44	36 to 44	22 to 26	±2·5
Alkalosis	More than 7·44	Less than 36	More than 26	More than +2·5

FIG. 35

Blood gas levels for arterial blood after Astrup. In practice the results are interpreted by first looking at the pH then referring to the Pco_2 to determine if the disturbance is respiratory. If the Pco_2 is normal then the base excess value is examined to determine the degree of metabolic upset. The standard bicarbonate figure is of less importance. e.g. If the arterial pH is 7.29, then acidosis is present. The Pco_2 is found to be 68 mm. Hg. and the base excess +2 mEq./1. The diagnosis is respiratory acidosis.

Standard bicarbonate measurement has one drawback, however, it does not give directly, in mEq./litre of blood, the amount of fixed acid or base causing a change in the base content of a blood sample. An additional term, " *base excess* " is helpful in determining these accumulated amounts of acid or base. If the normal value is zero then positive values signify an excess of base in the blood while negative values reflect a deficit of base, i.e. an excess of acid (Figs. 34 and 35).

In surgical practice, it has become more important to know the condition of the patient's respiratory system before anaesthesia and surgery are embarked upon. If the simple tests mentioned above were used more frequently pre-operatively many post-operative problems would be avoided. The tests are also a useful guide to the efficacy of any pre-operative drug therapy or physiotherapy which may be prescribed for the patient.

CHAPTER VI

INTRAVENOUS THERAPY

The ability to set up an intravenous infusion quickly and confidently under any circumstances is a great asset in any doctor and is particularly valuable to the anaesthetist who may have to do so sometimes under very difficult conditions. Provided there is no contra-indication and adequate assistance is available during anaesthesia, it is often easier to set up a drip after anaesthesia has been induced as the veins dilate and the procedure is not painful to the patient.

THE CHOICE OF INFUSION FLUID

The choice of infusion fluid depends on the indications for the infusion.

1. Glucose in Distilled Water

When an infusion is set up at the beginning of an operation so that an open vein will be available if blood is required during surgery or when the need is to infuse fluid without the addition of electrolytes, a solution of 5 per cent. glucose in sterile water may be used. Stronger solutions of glucose, 10 per cent. or even 50 per cent. may be used where calories are required but these are irritant and the infusion should take place only into a large vein. A long polythene cannula is used and particularly in the case of 50 per cent. glucose, transfused normally in cases of renal failure, the infusion should be into the vena cava. Laevulose solution is preferred by some clinicians as providing more calories and producing a lower incidence of phlebo-thrombosis in a long running infusion.

2. Electrolytes (Fig. 36)

Electrolytes such as sodium, potassium and chloride ions are given where electrolytic deficiency is found. Thus when there is loss of electrolyte as in prolonged vomiting, prolonged aspiration of stomach contents or reduced ingestion of fluids, careful observation of the electrolyte intake and output must be undertaken. This is done by daily measuring the electrolyte levels in the blood and calculating the requirements for the next 24 hours. It should be stressed that with the range of stock bottles and ampoules available nowadays replacement therapy should be a fairly exact science and no longer a matter of guesswork.

The use of mixed solutions of electrolytes such as Ringer lactate, containing sodium, potassium, calcium chloride and lactate in predetermined doses, is generally inferior to a regime calculated for each individual patient.

The practice of administering such fluids intravenously to all patients undergoing surgery because they will have been deprived of oral fluid for some 24 hours must also be carefully considered. The metabolic response to operation includes water and sodium retention and increased potassium loss. The duration of these changes ranges from 1-6 days. Over-enthusiastic administration of intravenous fluids may worsen this situation.

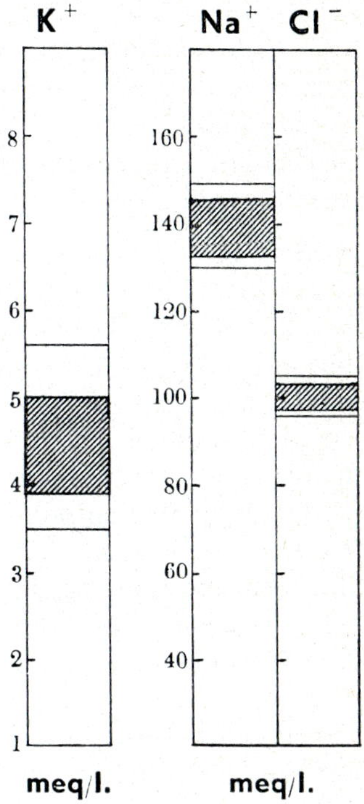

FIG. 36

A useful chart for recording the serum electrolyte levels. Levels which fall within the hatched area are normal, those in the small segments beyond may be normal, while values outside these limits are abnormal.

3. Blood

Normally blood is transfused when blood has been lost. It may be given pre-operatively to correct anaemia. In this case packed cells are often used but whole blood may be infused slowly where packed cells are not readily available. To counteract acute haemorrhage, however, whole blood, correctly grouped and cross-matched, is normally used. On occasion a proportion of the measured blood loss may be replaced by the use of a physiologically balanced electrolyte solution, e.g. Ringer lactate. When an anaesthetist commences the administration of blood during anaesthesia he must ensure that the bottles of blood being transfused are those which have been previously grouped and cross-matched for this particular patient. Very careful checking of the name and group on the bottle with those on the patient's case sheet is essential to ensure that no accidents take place. This is particularly important during anaesthesia when transfusion reactions are more difficult to recognise.

4. Plasma

Plasma may be transfused while blood is being obtained and cross-matched. This will restore the circulating volume but not replace the oxygen carrying capacity of the blood which has been lost. In addition, in patients who are hypo-volaemic and in electrolyte imbalance, plasma may be used to expand the circulatory volume and ensure adequate renal perfusion before administering aqueous electrolyte solutions. Even when plasma has been obtained from small pools of donors there remains the risk of transmitting serum hepatitis. This may vary from a minor upset in liver function to severe jaundice and may prejudice the life of a seriously ill patient. For this reason among others plasma substitutes have been developed. In some centres the administration of serum albu-men has replaced the use of whole plasma, as the hazards of hepatitis and other reactions are associated with the globulin fraction in the plasma.

5. Plasma Substitutes

A plasma substitute such as Macrodex may be given if blood or plasma are not readily available. This is a sugar solution containing large molecules (average molecular weight 70,000) with high osmotic pressure which acts as a plasma expander. A reduction in post-operative phlebothrombosis is also claimed where Macrodex has been given during and after operation. A further substance which may be used as a blood substitute is Rheomacrodex, a solution of smaller molecular weight (average molecular weight—40,000). It will restore the blood volume and in some cases the blood pressure and may increase renal output by reducing viscosity after a considerable amount of blood has been given. While it does not restore oxygen carrying capacity to the blood, by reducing the viscosity of the blood it increases blood flow and tissue perfusion and may thus increase the oxygenation of the tissues. Where blood has not been lost and only a small amount of fluid is required, Rheomacrodex or Macrodex, being much cheaper than blood, may be the agent of choice.

6. Sodium Bicarbonate Solution

In certain circumstances after anaesthesia and surgery and indeed before either, acidosis may be present. We will later discuss the problems of respiratory acidosis in which the pH is low and the Pa_{CO_2} is high. However, we are also concerned with metabolic acidosis and in this case the pH is low, the Pa_{CO_2} is low or normal and the standard bicarbonate and base excess levels measured in the blood are low. In these circumstances an infusion of sodium bicarbonate solution is useful and restores the pH and bicarbonate levels to normal. A chart showing the blood gas changes to be expected in acidosis and alkalosis both of respiratory and metabolic origin may be seen in Chapter V at page 72. The ' standard bicarbonate " is quoted in terms of mEq./litre as is the " base excess ". When metabolic acidosis is detected it is usual to calculate the bicarbonate requirement by multiplying the body weight in kilos, by a figure of 0·3 and multiplying the answer by the base excess. This figure gives the number of mEq. of sodium bicarbonate which are required to restore the standard bicarbonate and pH to normal. Another useful guide is to consider small patients as having 10 litres of total body fluid, medium sized patients about 12 litres and large patients about 15 litres of body fluid. The 10, 12 or 15 are multiplied by the base excess to find the number of mEq. of sodium bicarbonate to be administered. This rough guide is useful as it is very often in patients who have not been weighed, e.g. emergencies, that the acidosis is found.

Metabolic acidosis is frequently found in patients in whom the peripheral circulation has been inadequate for some time, e.g. perforated duodenal ulcer or coronary thrombosis. Anaerobic respiration in the tissues results in production of acid metabolites which are flushed into the general circulation when the regional perfusion is improved by appropriate treatment.

Metabolic acidosis may also be expected in patients who have been losing alkaline fluid such as bile, by aspiration, by a fistula or through a drainage tube. During operation patients may develop a metabolic acidosis where the peripheral circulation is impaired for a considerable period and subsequently dilates with release of acid metabolites into the circulation. This process is seen classically in patients during cardiopulmonary bypass and hypothermia. Here, careful biochemical control is undertaken during the operation and the pH level is kept near normality. Administration of large quantities of stored blood, which has a low pH, also results in the immediate production of metabolic acidosis and it is wise in such circumstances to administer at least 100 mEq. of sodium bicarbonate after each four pints of blood.

7. Intravenous Feeding

In some patients it is necessary to provide not only fluid but calorie requirements by the intravenous route for a considerable period. Special fluids are available which allow adequate calories to be given in relatively low fluid volumes. Preparations of amino-acids for intravenous use are also available (see p. 185).

APPARATUS AND TECHNIQUE

THE CHOICE OF APPARATUS with which to set up the infusion is of importance. The container of the infusion fluid may be a bottle, a flask or a disposable plastic pack. The choice of administration set will also depend on what is supplied in each hospital, though plastic disposable sets are now almost universally used. There is, however, a wide range of needles and cannulae available for use with the administration set.

A needle is supplied with each infusion set. While this is no doubt the easiest to insert into the vein it has many disadvantages from the point of view of the anaesthetist. If the drip is set up in the ward, the patient transported to the theatre, on to the operating table and then returned to his bed, there is a high probability that the needle will pierce the vein and the fluid will run into the tissues. For this reason it is common nowadays to use some form of cannula.

There are a number of cannulae available, metal being largely superseded by plastic types. Two of the more commonly used are illustrated at Figures 37 and 38. Both contain an inner metal needle and an outer plastic cannula. The combined unit is inserted into the vein and the needle then withdrawn leaving the blunt cannula free in the vein. These units represent an excellent compromise between a needle which is easier to insert but easy also to displace during movement and a plain cannula which requires the vein to be exposed and ligated before it can be inserted.

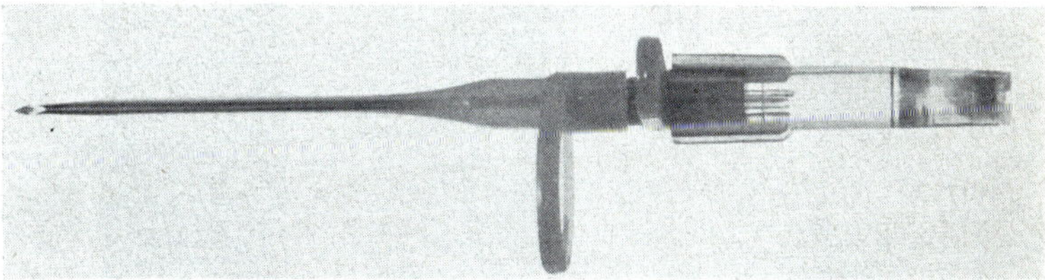

A

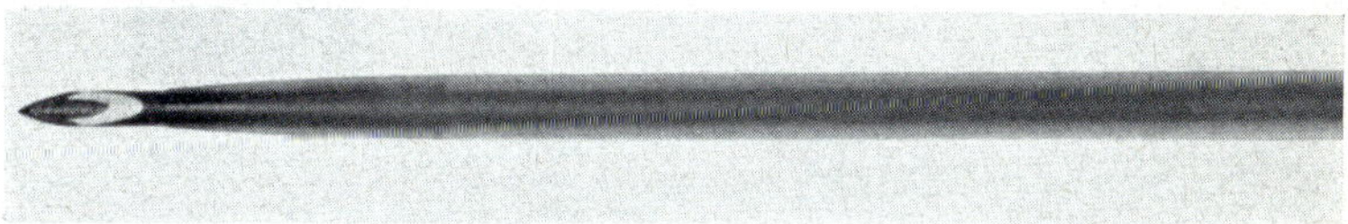

B

FIG. 37

The Braunula complete (A), and showing the needle projecting beyond the plastic cannula (B).

If difficulty is experienced in inserting the combined unit through the skin, a small incision with a Hagedorn needle may first be made or a drop of sterile lubricant applied to the tip of the needle.

These cannulae, though most frequently used for intravenous infusions, may be used for repeated injections or sampling from within a vessel. In this case a sterile rubber capped plug is inserted into the end of the cannula. For this latter purpose, that is repeated intravenous injections, special needles such as shown at Figures 39 and 40 may also be used.

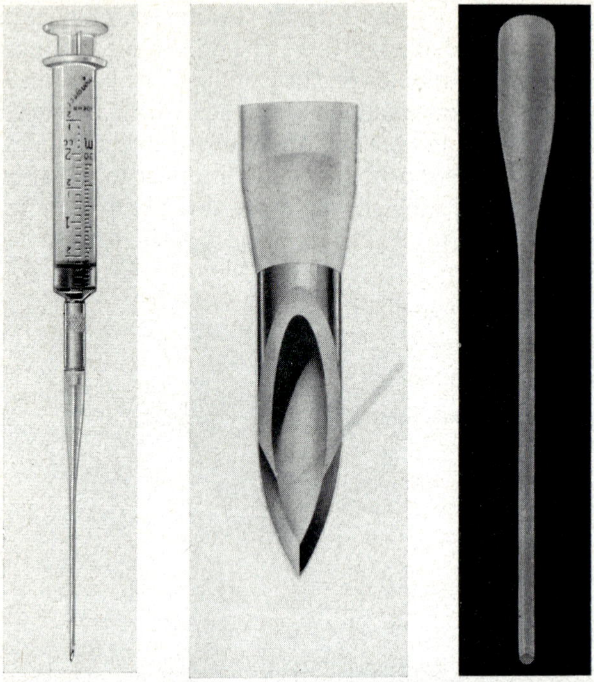

A B C

FIG. 38

The Medicut Cannula. (A) shows the syringe, needle and cannula assembled for venepuncture. (B) shows the tapered cannula closely fitting the needle. (C) shows the blunt cannula which remains in the vein when the needle and syringe are withdrawn.
Long polypropylene cannulae are available for use in conjunction with this set. When inserted through C they may be used to deliver irritant solutions into large veins or to measure the central venous pressure.

In infants a finer needle with a polythene tube extension may be inserted in a convenient scalp vein (Fig. 41).

Longer polythene cannulae may be used for long continued infusions. These should be fed through one of the short polythene cannulae described above and not through a metal needle. Many mishaps have occurred when combined units of the long cannula and metal needle have been used, where the cannula was severed by the sharp edge of the needle. New units

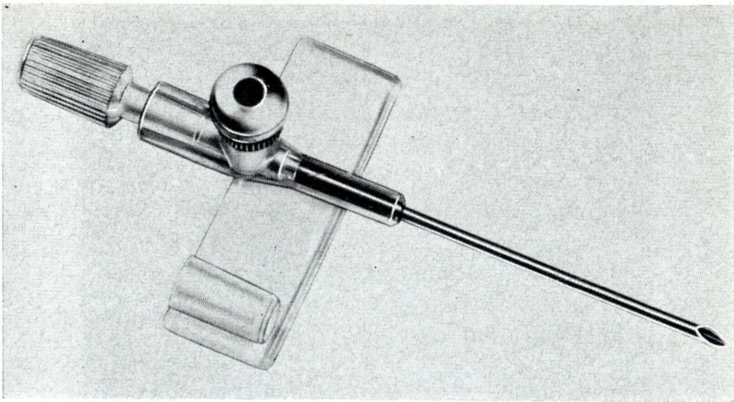

FIG. 39
The Viggo Needle. Injections may be made through the rubber diaphragm on the top of the needle. The plastic plug in the hub of the needle may be removed and injections or infusions delivered by this route.

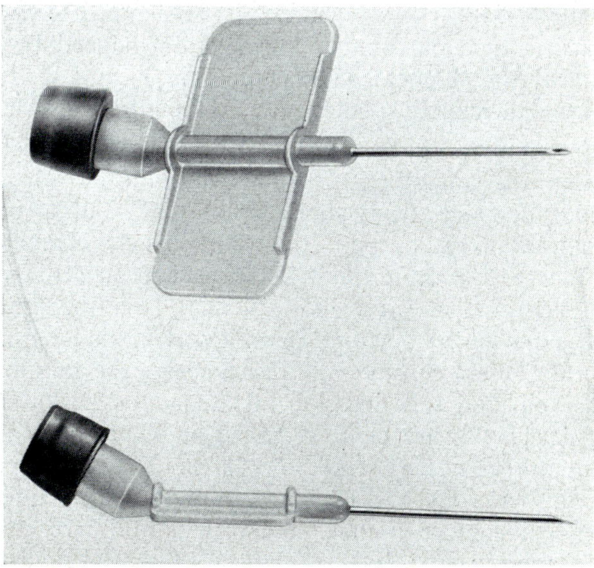

FIG. 40
The Armoven Needle. Injections may be given through the rubber diaphragm on the hub of the needle.

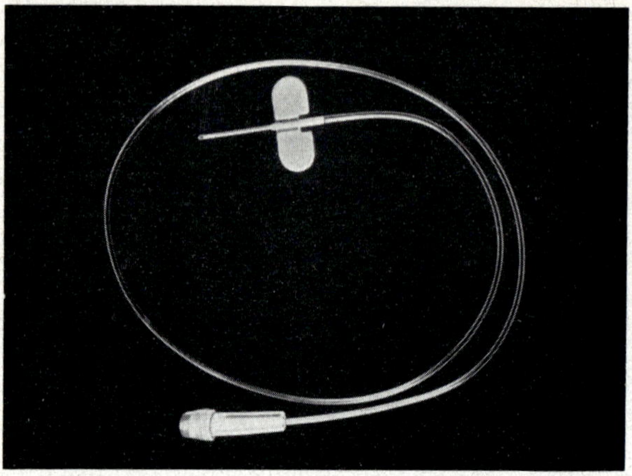

FIG. 41
Paediatric Scalp Vein Needle.

have been introduced whereby the benefits of the long polythene cannulae can be obtained without the hazards described (see Chapter XIX).

A further type of cannula normally introduced by direct exposure of the vein is a tapered polythene cannula. It is of wide bore and may be used for fast running infusions into the saphenous vein.

Usually, the anaesthetist requires an infusion which will run rapidly for a relatively short period, that is, up to perhaps 24 hours. For this purpose the short plastic cannulae are ideal. Where, however, an infusion is expected to run for several days and speed is not essential then the long thin polythene one is very suitable. Here, however, the long, narrow bore tubing offers considerable resistance to the flow of fluid into the vein and thus infusion takes place at a slower rate. Where electrolytes are being replaced or where more irritant solutions are being delivered into larger, free running veins these considerations are not important. Nutrient infusions, however, being more viscous, should be administered through the wide tapering cannula.

THE SITE CHOSEN for the venepuncture is of considerable importance (Fig. 42). The veins of the antecubital fossa although very tempting and usually of considerable size are less suitable for infusion during an operation. Movement of the elbow tends to displace the point or impede the flow through the cannula and other sites are preferred. Among these are the veins available at the wrist and on the back of the hand.

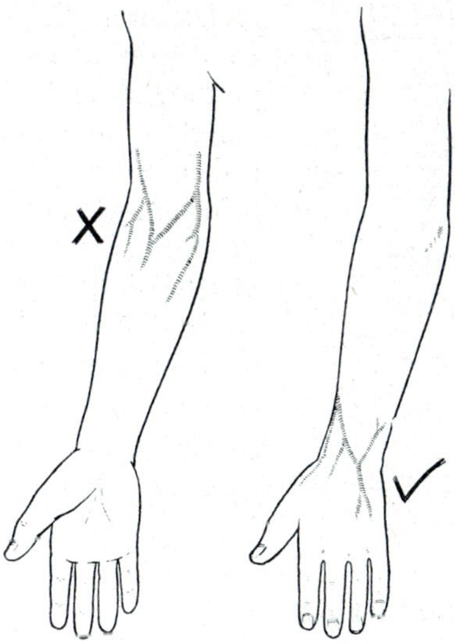

FIG. 42
Possible sites for setting up infusions. If the veins round the wrist and the back of the hand are chosen, greater mobility of the limb is possible without dislodging the needle or cannula.

An infusion inserted here is readily accessible to the anaesthetist during the operation and injections can be made into it without disturbing the surgical procedure. The wrist can be easily splinted, if necessary, although often this is unnecessary and the patient after operation can be allowed full movement of the hand, provided care is taken to fix the cannula well as it enters the skin.

Normally in a right handed person it is preferable to set up an infusion in the left hand as this allows the patient the use of the hand which is of most value to him. This is a point often overlooked.

Where possible the leg should not be used for infusions as there is a considerable incidence of phlebitis following infusions, particularly of irritant solutions or those which have run for some considerable time (over 48 hours). As the venous blood flow is less rapid than in the arms and as the leg veins are of larger size, leg vein thrombosis is more likely to occur and is more liable to be followed by serious consequences such as pulmonary embolism.

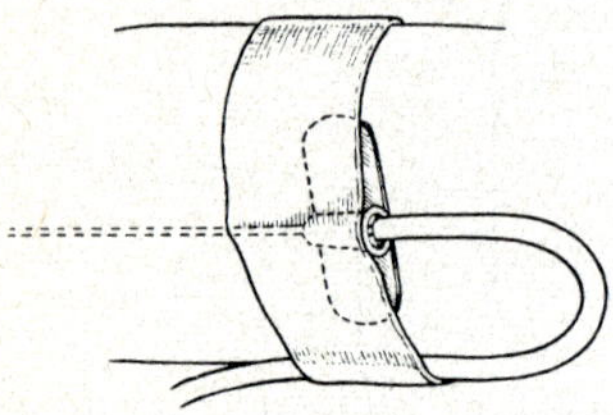

FIG. 43

If the apparatus is secured in the manner shown, traction on the tubing is less likely to dislodge the cannula.

Before embarking upon the task of setting up an intravenous infusion, the doctor should ensure that everything from the bottle of infusion fluid down to the swabs and tape to secure the cannula are immediately at hand. It is wise to secure a loop of the giving set at the site of connection to the cannula to prevent any pull on the giving set dislodging the cannula (Fig. 43).

Transfusion under Pressure

Under certain circumstances it may be desirable to administer fluids, particularly blood, under pressure.

Two methods of delivering blood under pressure are shown. The first, Martin's type pump (Fig. 44) is clamped to the drip stand and the tubing from the giving set fed through it. As the handle of the pump is turned the rollers press the fluid down through the tubing and thus force it into the patient's vein. A second method of administration of fluids under pressure is shown in Figure 45. This is a special giving set made of polythene and a second chamber containing a ball valve is compressed to force the fluid into the patient.

Temperature of Blood

Blood stored in a refrigerator will be transfused at a temperature below that of the body—the difference varying with the time lapse between removal and transfusion and the rate of transfusion. With slow transfusions of relatively small amounts

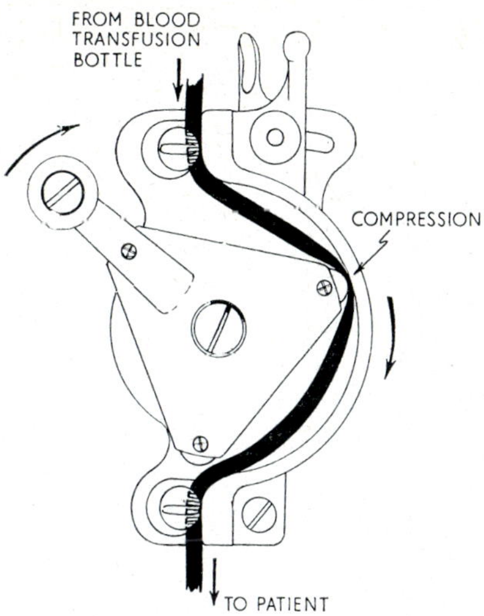

FIG. 44

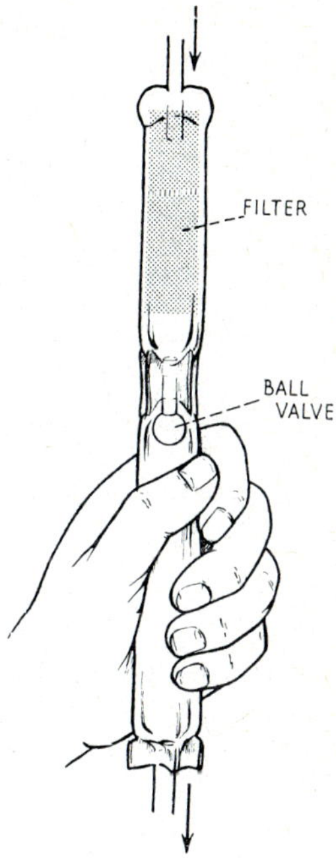

FIG. 45

FIG. 44. The Martin Pump. When the handle is turned in the direction indicated, the rollers force blood down the tubing to the patient.

FIG. 45. A pressure transfusion set. The lower chamber is allowed to fill with blood by compressing and releasing it. The ball valve floats on the blood and when the full chamber is again compressed the ball occludes the upper outlet and blood is forced down the tubing to the patient.

of blood the lower temperature of the blood is of little consequence. Where, however, large quantities of cold blood are transfused rapidly, a severe fall in body temperature may result leading to a cardiac arrest. Steps must therefore be taken to warm the blood to body temperature. This may be done by warming the bottle or container or by passing the blood through a coil immersed in warm water en route to the patient (Fig. 46).

The administration of calcium as the chloride or gluconate is also essential when massive blood transfusions are given.

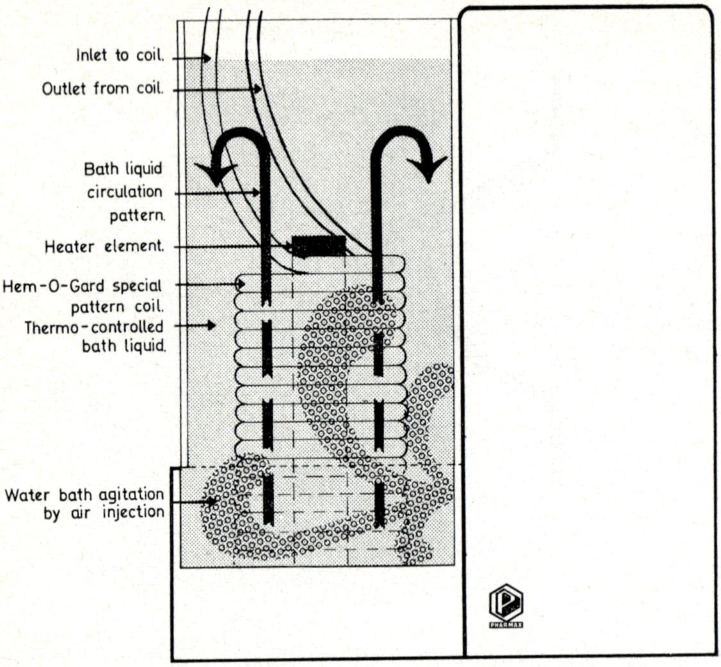

FIG. 46

Schematic diagram of operation of Hem-O Gard blood warming equipment.

BLOOD LOSS ESTIMATIONS

It is often not clear when to begin blood replacement and when to discontinue it. Ideally, of course, blood volume measurements should be undertaken and haematocrit readings may also be useful. Often, however, such measurements are impracticable and the value of haemoglobin levels or haematocrit readings will depend to a large extent on the degree of haemo-concentration or haemo-dilution present. It is thus important to consider the clinical indications for transfusion and the indications that transfusion has been adequate (Fig. 47).

It is possible by weighing the swabs which have been used during operation and comparing them with dry swabs to estimate the amount of blood which has been lost. It is also possible to wash the blood from the swabs and by using a colorimeter to measure the quantity lost.

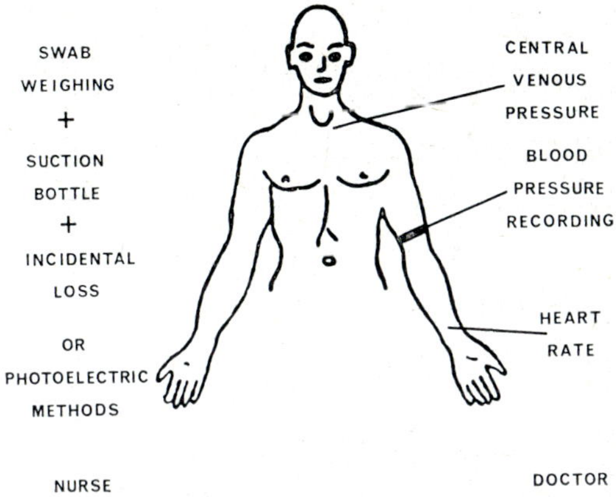

FIG. 47
Methods of assessing blood loss. The methods in which the nurse assists are shown on the left of the diagram.

When blood is lost certain physiological responses take place. In the first instance the peripheral circulation is reduced and the blood flow through the extremities, as measured by the plethysmograph, falls. Only when this process can no longer compensate for the haemorrhage does the heart rate start to rise. When the increase in heart rate is no longer adequate to compensate for the blood loss the blood pressure falls. This is shown in Figure 48.

Where blood loss is overt and appears likely to continue it is desirable that replacement should be commenced before the onset of tachycardia and certainly before the blood pressure has fallen markedly. Similarly, provided other causes of tachycardia and hypotension can be excluded, it is desirable to continue the transfusion until the blood pressure and the pulse rate have returned to normal. Some indication of the adequacy of blood replacement can be gained by observing the filling of the neck veins when the patient is lying flat or with the head slightly raised. The central venous pressure may also be more accurately measured by means of a cannula passed into the superior or inferior vena cava and attached to a saline manometer. A stable central venous pressure is another indication that replacement of blood loss has been adequate (see p. 185).

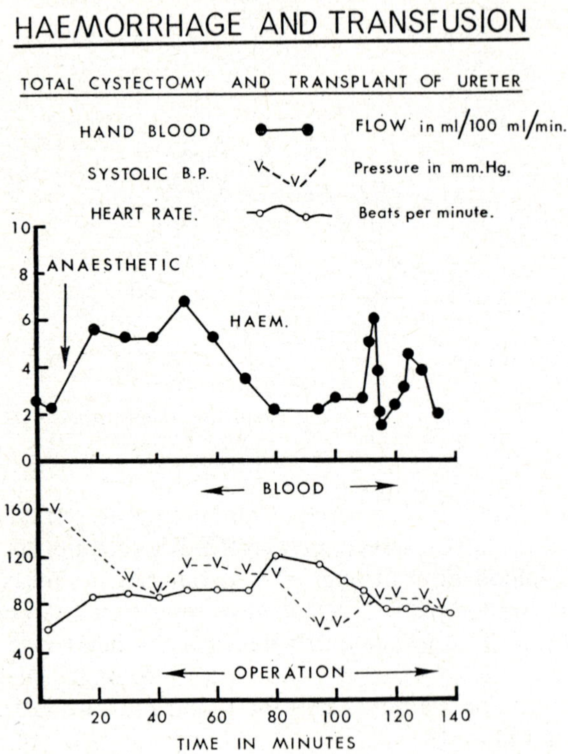

FIG. 48

The effects of haemorrhage and transfusion on blood flow, blood pressure and heart rate during surgery.

Blood volume and haematocrit measurements on the day following operation will indicate whether the blood volume and haemoglobin levels have been restored to normal.

Blood volume measurements, using either a dye dilution technique or dilution method with radioactive isotopes, can be performed in theatre and during certain operations the blood volume is regularly monitored in this way. During the repair of congenital cardiac defects in children this method is vital.

It is not possible in this chapter to deal extensively with all the problems associated with intravenous therapy. Remember when setting up an infusion to think what you are trying to replace and what is the most logical way of replacing it. Never give blood if it is not indicated and conversely do not hesitate to use blood where it is indicated, bearing in mind the replacement of blood volume and of haemoglobin with its oxygen carrying capacity. Where possible measure the blood loss. Blood volume measurements are an obvious guide to the amount of blood or blood substitute to be administered and the haematocrit will give some indication of the haemoglobin levels. Knowledge of the electrolyte values in the blood will allow the correct amount and type of electrolyte to be replaced. In the same way acid-base measurements allow acidosis or alkalosis to be corrected.

In transfusing small children, note that their blood volume is approximately 50 ml. per pound of body weight and that a pint of blood to a small child may represent a considerable proportion of the normal blood volume. Try neither to under transfuse nor to over transfuse. On the one hand an extra load is thrown on the circulation, as the heart has to beat faster to compensate for the deficiency in blood volume; on the other hand the administration of excessive quantities of blood will also throw an additional strain on the heart.

The control of intravenous infusions in general is the place for co-operation between surgeon, anaesthetist and biochemist. Remember that if the need for large quantities of blood is anticipated the blood bank must be warned in plenty of time as there may be difficulty in providing your requirements at a moment's notice.

CHAPTER VII

THE ADMINISTRATION OF A GENERAL ANAESTHETIC

An anaesthetic can be divided into induction and maintenance. These two may merge imperceptibly or there may be a fairly sharp demarcation line between them. Induction of anaesthesia is considered to last from the moment when the anaesthetic is commenced until the requisite level of anaesthesia has been achieved for whatever operation is contemplated. This may take a few minutes or a considerable time, depending upon the method chosen and on the skill of the anaesthetist.

INDUCTION OF ANAESTHESIA

Induction of anaesthesia is usually achieved in one of two ways, by intravenous injection of suitable agents or by inhalation of gaseous anaesthetics or vapours of volatile anaesthetic liquids. Before selecting a method for any case several questions must be answered.

1. What is the safest method of induction?
2. What is most pleasant for the patient?
3. Which is the easiest and most practicable method under the circumstances?

The safety of each method lies in the avoidance of the complications associated with induction of anaesthesia. These may be (1) regurgitation as the oesophageal sphincter relaxes, (2) hypoxia associated with coughing, bucking or laryngeal spasm, (3) respiratory depression, (4) fall in blood pressure resulting in cardiac insufficiency.

Many of these may be avoided by slow careful injection but apart from the hypoxia due to coughing, straining and laryngeal spasm, the other dangers are more liable to accompany rapid induction of anaesthesia with an intravenous agent. The patient retains most of his protective reflexes during an inhalational induction and, should he vomit, can cough and clear his airway, provided he is in reasonable health. This may not be so in a frail patient.

1. Intravenous Induction of Anaesthesia

The drugs normally employed are considered in the section on pharmacology. Here we will describe only a thiopentone induction.

This drug should be made up in a 2·5 per cent. rather than a 5 per cent. solution as it has been shown that accidental injection of thiopentone into an artery is more likely to be followed by serious complications, such as intravascular thrombosis and gangrene, where a 5 per cent. solution has been used. In addition the use of the more dilute solution is less liable to lead to accidental overdosage.

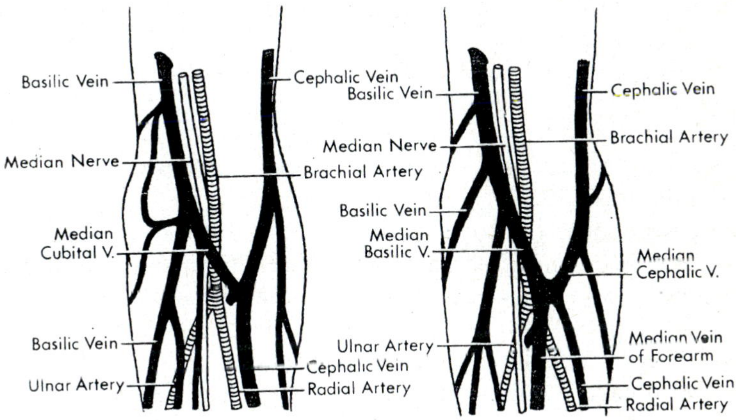

FIG. 49

Showing arrangement of veins in region of cubital fossa (left arm).

Showing an alternative and frequently seen arrangement of veins in the same region (left arm).

A suitable vein should be sought for and exposed and the arm compressed proximally to it. The vessel is then palpated to ensure that it is not pulsating and the radial pulse also checked to see that arterial pulsation has not been obliterated by the compression of the arm. A vein on the dorsum of the hand is commended as this is the site least likely to lead to accidental intra-arterial injection. If such a vein is not easily accessible then one on the lateral aspect of the antecubital fossa should be selected. The use of the medial side of the antecubital fossa should be avoided whenever possible because of the risk of injection into an artery and in addition the median nerve is very vulnerable at this site (Fig. 49).

After these precautions have been observed the needle is inserted and blood aspirated to make sure that the needle is indeed in the vein. The colour of the aspirated blood will depend on several factors and in a well sedated patient little oxygen is removed from the peripheral blood in the hand and therefore even venous blood from the back of the hand may be bright red. There should however be no signs of active pulsation of the blood into the syringe at any time. Pressure on the arm above the vein is now released and 1-2 ml. of solution are injected.

Thereafter the injection is halted and a few moments allowed for the drug to circulate. The patient is then asked whether he feels any pain in the limb at or below the point of injection. This is an essential precaution (p. 260).

If this test has been negative and the patient has not complained of any pain, a further 2-3 ml. should be injected after which a further pause is allowed and a further 2-3 ml. of solution injected.

It is essential that one should have no fixed ideas as to the dose of thiopentone to be given before starting the injection. Rather should one inject small quantities at suitable intervals until the patient loses consciousness. If the patient is ill and has a slow circulation then longer pauses will be required between each 2-3 ml. to allow the drug to circulate. The total dose of drug required to produce unconsciousness may vary widely, the ill, debilitated patient requiring perhaps 100 mg., the large alcoholic labourer taking little short of 1 G. It is a popular practice to ask the patient to count and when he ceases counting it is assumed that he has fallen asleep. However, some patients can continue counting in an automatic fashion beyond the point at which they can respond sensibly to questions asked in conversation. Many anaesthetists therefore prefer rather to speak to the patient and to note the point at which he ceases to answer or take part in the conversation.

When sleep has ensued, it is normally advisable to cease the injection of thiopentone as the drug is intended only to induce sleep and adds little to the further conduct of the anaesthetic. The induction is continued by administration of nitrous oxide and 33 per cent. oxygen and if necessary a volatile agent such as trichloroethylene (Trilene), halothane or ether. If Trilene is chosen it is added to the gas and oxygen mixture by slowly advancing the lever on the side of the bottle until it is fully open but the plunger is never depressed into the bottle. If halothane is chosen increments of 0·5 per cent. at a time are added to reach perhaps 3-4 per cent. depending on the response of the patient, but this concentration will be maintained only for a short time. If it is decided to use ether, which is more irritant, then addition of the ether to the mixture will be achieved by flicking on and off the lever at the side of the bottle with a suitable interval, say four breaths, between each movement until no reaction to the ether is obtained. Thereafter the lever will be slowly advanced up the scale again allowing four clear breaths between each movement.

2. Inhalational Induction of Anaesthesia

This may be achieved in one of several ways.

Until recently inhalational anaesthesia was often induced with gaseous mixtures containing less than 20 per cent. oxygen —sometimes none at all. This technique was used because it was considered to provide a more rapid induction of anaesthesia which was more pleasant for the patient and avoided some of the complications of the " excitement stage " of Guedel's classification (p. 95). Not only did these techniques produce potentially dangerous hypoxia but inhalation of gaseous mixtures containing at least 20 per cent. oxygen have been shown not to prolong induction of anaesthesia significantly. Two techniques will be described.

In the first the patient is asked to breathe a mixture of nitrous oxide (7 litres) and oxygen (3 litres). This is continued until consciousness is lost as evidenced by loss of eyelash reflex or the onset of " automatic " respiration, regular in rate or depth. A volatile agent, usually halothane, is now added in gradually increasing percentage until the required level of anaesthesia is reached.

When introducing the other volatile agents the same considerations apply as after a thiopentone induction. In robust patients some anaesthetists favour the addition of 0·5 per cent. halothane to the inhaled mixture after about 20 breaths even in the absence of signs of unconsciousness.

Bourne has described a technique by which a six litre reservoir bag is filled with a mixture containing 50 per cent. each of cyclopropane and oxygen. The patient again breathes from a close fitting mask and rebreathes into the bag. Consciousness is lost after not more than 12 breaths and anaesthesia may be continued with nitrous oxide and oxygen and a supplement. Alternatively if the cyclopropane/oxygen mixture is inhaled for one minute, satisfactory operating conditions will persist for a further 1½ minutes.

3. Pre-oxygenation

The techniques described are usually satisfactory for adults in normal health. In patients with a poor cardio-respiratory reserve or a potentially full stomach (see p. 55) or where difficulty is anticipated during induction, a reserve of oxygen in the blood is invaluable. If 100 per cent. oxygen is breathed for five minutes a large part of the nitrogen in the lungs will be washed out and replaced by oxygen and the arterial oxygen tension raised by up to 500 per cent.

With this reserve in hand coughing or laryngeal spasm which might otherwise produce dangerous hypoxia may be safely dealt with in time or a difficult tracheal intubation may be accomplished without hypoxia.

It is wise to practise the technique of pre-oxygenation for, although it is possibly unnecessary for many cases, it is always a valuable safeguard.

As we have now induced anaesthesia to a light level, administration of inhalational agents will continue until the anaesthesia is considered to be deep enough for the operation to be commenced. This will obviously vary with the particular operation and the degree of muscular relaxation required for its performance. No mention has so far been made of the use of muscle relaxants and these will be considered separately, as they involve the problems of assisted or controlled ventilation.

Before we can rationally decide when to reduce the concentration of volatile anaesthetics and judge that the patient is at a level of anaesthesia adequate for any particular operation, we must consider the signs of anaesthesia, as they will give us some guide as to the level of unconsciousness which has been or must be attained.

THE SIGNS OF ANAESTHESIA

The stages and signs of anaesthesia, as normally described and taught are those formulated by Guedel and apply to ether anaesthesia after atropine premedication. A modified table of Guedel's signs is shown in Figure 50.

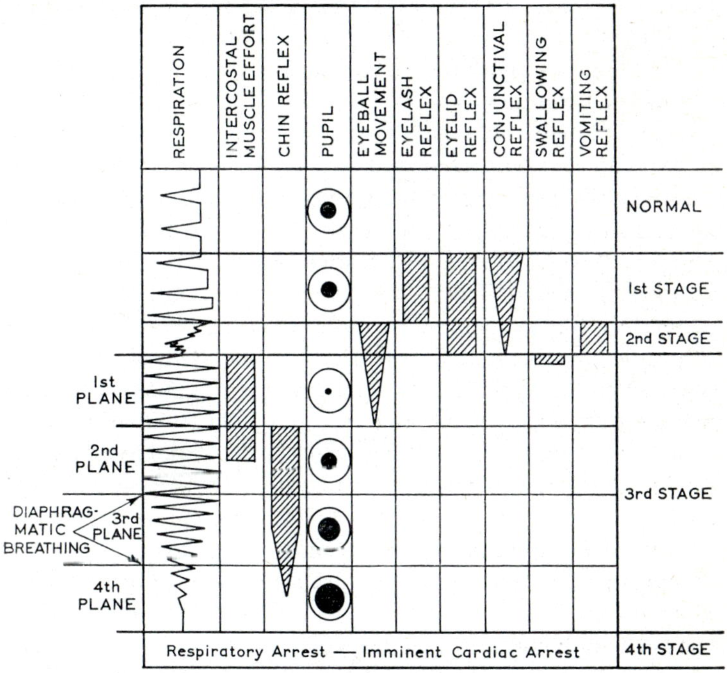

FIG. 50

Stages and Signs of Anaesthesia (after Guedel 1937). Many of these signs may be used to estimate the depth of unconsciousness resulting from other causes, e.g. head injuries.

Many students are rather puzzled to see that the classical stages and signs about which they have read are not in evidence when modern anaesthetic techniques are used. There are, however, good reasons for this and we have discussed earlier the division of anaesthesia into its three parts—sleep, analgesia and muscular relaxation. It is this division of anaesthesia into its component parts and the use of specific drugs to produce them which has revolutionised anaesthesia but it also means that one can, for instance, produce apnoea, which does not occur until Stage IV in Guedel's classification, by the use of a muscle relaxant without having produced either unconsciousness or indeed any analgesia. Similarly, it is possible, by rapid injection of a barbiturate, to produce apnoea and yet have a patient who will respond to a painful stimulus. It is for this reason that using present day anaesthetic techniques, the anaesthetist must depend on other signs to identify depth of anaesthesia.

A. Loss of Consciousness

When thiopentone is used it is not difficult to tell when the patient has lost consciousness. A method has already been described whereby the patient may be asked to count or is engaged in conversation and when the conversation ceases the patient is deemed to have lost consciousness. Using inhalational methods the distinction is not quite so clear but the onset of automatic, that is regular, respiration is a sure sign that consciousness has been lost. In addition the loss of the eyelid reflex, when the eyelash is stroked with the finger and the eyelid no longer closes, is a valuable guide to loss of consciousness. A further test which is valuable is to ask the patient to hold one arm in the air and when the arm falls to his side he is asleep.

When anaesthesia is continued with nitrous oxide, oxygen and a volatile supplement, the problem of the patient regaining consciousness during anaesthesia seldom arises. On rare occasions patients maintained on nitrous oxide, oxygen and a muscle relaxant may complain that they remember incidents during an operation. This is normally in circumstances where no sedative premedication has been used, a limited dose of thiopentone has been given for induction and anaesthesia has been maintained using nitrous oxide and more than 33 per cent. oxygen.

The use of hyoscine in premedication in place of atropine reduces this incidence of awareness during anaesthesia which occurs principally in obstetric practice.

The routine use of a supplementary volatile agent with nitrous oxide and oxygen should abolish this hazard in surgical practice but is associated with a slower recovery of consciousness.

The return of the eyelash reflex and movements of the eyelids and eyebrows in a paralysed patient should suggest that the patient requires more anaesthetic supplementation.

B. Assessment of Analgesia

As before, when anaesthesia is maintained by inhalation of ether it is possible to gauge the depth of anaesthesia by using Guedel's signs. However, with other agents and particularly when respiration is assisted after administration of muscle relaxants, other signs must be sought for. These are in fact the normal physiological reactions of the conscious person to pain, modified according to the degree of analgesia present and whether or not a muscle relaxant has been used.

1. WITHDRAWAL FROM THE PAINFUL STIMULUS. This may take the form of gross movement, that is a hand may be withdrawn from the surgeon's knife or the patient may draw up his knee. Such gross movement will take place when the patient is much too light and a severe stimulus is being applied. When, however, the depth of anaesthesia is just insufficient for the operation to be performed and when a muscle relaxant has been used in some quantity then the reaction may be restricted to slight movement of the fingers and hand or wrinkling of the forehead.

2. PHONATION. Patients will normally cry out when hurt and if it is possible some attempt at phonation is usually made. This is obviously not possible when an endotracheal tube is in place.

3. IRREGULAR RESPIRATION OR BREATH HOLDING may be signs of inadequate analgesia for the operation being performed. Laryngeal stridor may be included under this heading.

4. A further group of signs are associated with the liberation of adrenal hormones which are part of the " fight and flight " reaction.

(*a*) THE SKIN is seen to be pale, cold and sweating.

(*b*) THE HEART RATE is increased.

(*c*) THE BLOOD PRESSURE rises.

5. Another sign which is often found is LACHRYMATION.

These signs may be found at the beginning of the operation when the surgeon's skin incision is made, during operation if the anaesthetic becomes too light or in operations where painful stimuli are inflicted at intervals. They are an indication to increase the depth of anaesthesia by increasing the concentration of the volatile agents which are being administered or if only nitrous oxide and oxygen are being administered, they are an indication for the addition of a volatile agent to the mixture. An alternative is to give small doses of narcotics e.g. pethidine (10-25 mg.) intravenously.

C. Is Muscular Relaxation Adequate?

The degree of muscular relaxation needed for any particular operation is a matter which can be decided by experience and a little foresight.

As before when using ether anaesthesia it is possible by looking for the signs in Guedel's classification to decide in what stage the patient is and therefore what degree of muscular relaxation may be expected. Careful observation of these signs during inhalational anaesthesia will ensure that the appropriate level of anaesthesia is maintained throughout.

Where minor procedures, such as the manipulation of a fracture, are to be carried out it is possible after anaesthesia has been induced to test the relaxation in the limb concerned. It must however be remembered that while a limb may be flaccid at rest, when painful manipulation is carried out the muscles may contract.

Where a muscle relaxant has been administered and ventilation is being controlled, it may be difficult for the anaesthetist to decide whether relaxation remains adequate. Although respiration may have been abolished by the original dose of muscle relaxant, in many cases, the fact that respiration has not restarted is not of itself a sufficient indication that relaxation remains complete. While ventilation is controlled the level of carbon dioxide in the blood may be reduced and, if there has been any central depression, by the use of narcotics in premedication, by thiopentone induction of anaesthesia or by the addition of volatile agents during the anaesthetic itself, this may keep the patient apnoeic after muscular relaxation has at least partially worn off. Some guides to the fact that relaxation is wearing off are as follows:—

1. The surgeon may complain that the patient is " tight ". This is not always a reliable guide as surgeons tend to differ in their estimation of what is adequate relaxation. On the other hand some surgeons, particularly when working with a junior anaesthetist, to spare him embarrassment, may not complain when the patient is indeed tight!

2. If the anaesthetist watches the operation wound in the abdomen he may see that bowel is being pushed out through the wound and that the peritoneum is retracted deep down into the wound or tears as the surgeon is stitching up.

3. If respiration is being controlled by manual compression of the reservoir bag, the anaesthetist may notice that the pressure required to inflate the lungs is increasing and that greater effort has to be used to inflate the lungs with the same volume of gases. If a mechanical ventilator is being used then it is possible that, to maintain the same tidal volume, a higher pressure is required or if the ventilator is set to deliver a constant pressure it is noticed that a smaller volume of gas is being delivered to the patient by the same pressure. This is due to returning tone in the muscles of the chest wall and upper abdomen.

4. If the anaesthetist does not appreciate that a higher inflation pressure is being used and unconsciously compensates by increasing the pressure in the bag he may notice that the blood pressure is falling without obvious reason. This is due to the increased intrathoracic pressure reducing the venous return and thus the cardiac output (see p. 179).

5. The patient may start to make respiratory efforts. Alternatively if central depression is marked he may cough.

When muscular relaxation is seen to be inadequate in this way, the anaesthetic is either deepened, if inhalation agents only are being used or, if muscle relaxants have been given, an appropriate supplementary dose of the relaxant agent is administered intravenously.

One must consider what signs are most likely to be shown by the patient under the circumstances of any given anaesthetic. If an opiate has been used in premedication and thiopentone has been given early in the anaesthetic, the patient's pupils are likely to be small throughout the anaesthetic in the absence of gross hypoxia or very severe painful stimuli. Similarly, when muscle relaxant drugs have been administered the eyeball will remain fixed while they are still acting.

Some anaesthetists consider that, provided the patient is adequately relaxed and hyperventilation is undertaken, the signs suggestive of inadequate analgesia are not of importance, as it has never been established that patients suffer in any way from operations carried out under such circumstances. It has indeed been shown that even under deeper levels of anaesthesia, where there are no outward signs that the patient is receiving painful stimuli, such stimuli in fact do reach the cerebral cortex and there is little indication that the patient is any the worse for this. The only way of blocking the passage of these impulses to the brain is to do so by regional techniques, that is blocking the impulse in its passage along nerves before they reach the spinal cord. It is however, felt by many people that since these signs are in the way of being manifestations of protective mechanisms in action it is advisable to administer further analgesic drugs to abolish them.

THE FURTHER MAINTENANCE AND CONCLUSION OF ANAESTHESIA

We have dealt at some length with the recognition of various signs during anaesthesia. If one understands what to look for and recognises the state in which the patient is during anaesthesia then appropriate action can be taken. Thus if the patient is inadequately anaesthetised, further increments of intravenous analgesic or volatile agents can be given: if he is inadequately relaxed again appropriate measures can be taken and where he is showing signs of inadequate respiration, this can be augmented. Similarly, by knowing under what circumstances complications are liable to occur many can be prevented and by early recognition of the complications which do arise, prompt treatment will ensure that anaesthesia continues smoothly.

We may, however, consider in further detail the administration of two types of anaesthetic.

Spontaneous Respiration with Inhalational Agents

Anaesthesia may be induced either by intravenous or inhalational methods as mentioned in the section on induction of anaesthesia. The patient will have been anaesthetised to the level appropriate for the particular operation and the anaesthetist will watch for the signs which indicate that this level has been reached. He will then keep a regular check on the signs of anaesthesia at the level which he has chosen and, provided they are maintained, a low concentration of vapour such as 0·5 per cent. to 1 per cent. halothane will suffice for a prolonged period. Towards the end of operation the level of anaesthesia may be lightened but the extent of this will depend on the depth to which anaesthesia has been carried and the nature of the operation. Thus if nitrous oxide/oxygen and ether have been given for an intra-abdominal procedure the ether can probably be discontinued when the peritoneum is closed. On the other hand if only light anaesthesia has been maintained with nitrous oxide/oxygen and halothane for a superficial operation it is probably necessary to continue the administration of halothane until shortly before the wound is closed, otherwise the patient will awaken before the operation is completed.

While it is desirable to have a patient regain consciousness within a few minutes of the termination of operation, it is a risky procedure to try to maintain a patient at a very light level of anaesthesia, since it is at this level that vomiting, coughing and laryngeal spasm are most prone to take place. Thus adequate anaesthesia should be maintained until one is in a position to deal with these conditions on emergence, without interrupting the course of the operation.

Controlled Ventilation using Muscle Relaxants

Anaesthesia will usually be induced by the use of an intravenous barbiturate and a muscle relaxant will be given to paralyse the patient. Thereafter an endotracheal tube will be passed and ventilation controlled by manual or mechanical means. During the anaesthetic, the signs of inadequate analgesia and inadequate respiration will be sought and the patient carefully observed to ensure that relaxation is adequate. Supplements of analgesic or relaxant drugs will be given on indication and these procedures will be continued throughout the operation. Once the peritoneum is closed, the patient, usually still apnoeic, will have to be prepared for the end of the operation and steps are now taken to restore spontaneous respiration.

If the muscle relaxant is still considered to be acting, and, if the peritoneum has been closed easily this will be so, the appropriate antagonist drug will be given. In the case of *d*-tubocurarine, gallamine, alcuronium or pancuronium this is neostigmine in a dose of up to 2·5 mg. intravenously. As this drug produces severe bradycardia, marked salivation and possibly bronchospasm, it is preceded by atropine, normally 1·2 mg., administered intravenously. Where large doses of relaxant have been given it may be necessary to give up to 5 mg. of neostigmine but this should seldom be required.

If spontaneous respiration does not follow the administration of these drugs, further steps will be decided upon, in the light of the possible causes of continued apnoea. If hyperventilation has been carried out throughout the operation many anaesthetists would administer carbon dioxide 5-10 per cent. for a limited number of breaths, say 10 to 20 ventilations. If this does not succeed in starting the patient breathing, then, at the end of operation when tracheo-bronchial suction is being performed, the passage of the catheter into the trachea or into the pharynx is often sufficient as a non-specific stimulus to start respiration. Alternatively, a small dose of intravenous nikethamide (Coramine) may provide the required stimulus. This should, however, rarely be necessary and it is also seldom necessary to give an antagonist to pethidine if it has been administered and even more rarely is an analeptic required in an attempt to correct barbiturate overdose.

Normally, when an endotracheal tube is in place, tracheobronchial suction, using a catheter, through the tube is undertaken to remove any bronchial secretions. In addition an intravenous dose of nikethamide (2-6 ml.) is useful particularly in patients who are known to have excessive bronchial secretions as the hyperventilation and coughing which follow enable these secretions to be delivered into the trachea and main bronchi, where they are accessible to suction. After suction through the endotracheal tube, the pharynx should be aspirated through a " whistle-tip " catheter before deflating the cuff on the endotracheal tube. Once the pharynx has been aspirated the same catheter should not be used again in the trachea, lest infection is introduced in this way. At this stage the patient may be transferred to a tilting trolley and placed on her side (Fig. 51).

When the anaesthetist is satisfied that the patient is recovering and is fit for return to the ward, she should be handed into the care of a responsible person. It is important

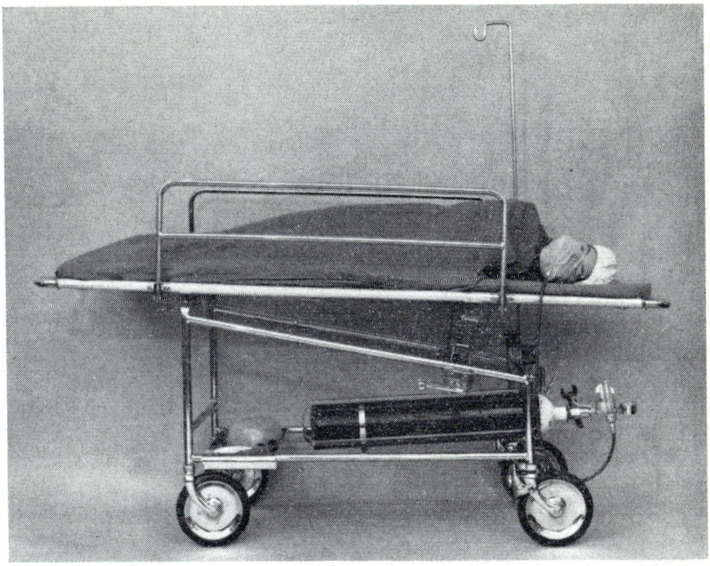

FIG. 51

Patient on tilting trolley awaiting transfer to the recovery room. The cylinder of oxygen is clearly seen and the mechanism for tilting with the handle in place is above the cylinder. The tray with instruments is shown on the left above the wheels.

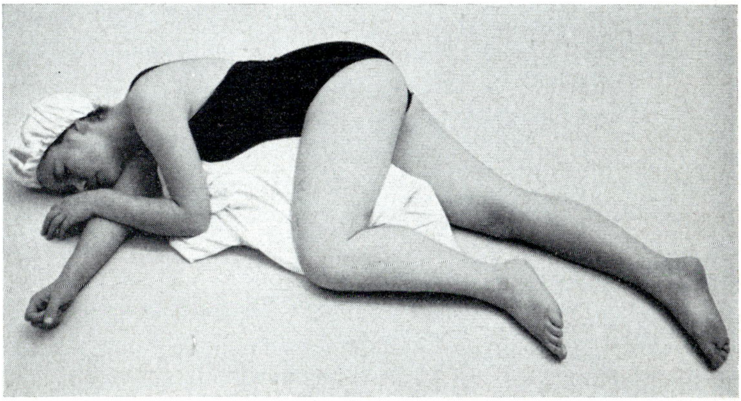

FIG. 52

The tonsillar position: the patient lies midway between the lateral and the prone positions, prevented from rolling face downwards by the pillow and the position of the arms and legs.

to remember that, until this is done, the responsibility for the patient's safety rests with the person who is giving the anaesthetic. A useful test at this stage, if muscle relaxant drugs have been given, is to ask the patient to put out her tongue. If she can do this and show that she is conscious and able to respond to simple instructions then she is in a safe state to return to the ward. When in doubt, the anaesthetist himself should see his patient safely back in bed and preferably in the tonsillar position (Fig. 52). In this position the tongue falls forward, the airway remains clear and if vomiting or regurgitation should occur the vomitus will flow away from the air passages (see p. 141). Never be rushed into starting another case before you are satisfied with the condition of the previous patient. A few minutes' lack of supervision at this stage may undo hours of careful work in the theatre.

CHAPTER VIII

ENDOTRACHEAL INTUBATION AND ENDOSCOPY

ENDOTRACHEAL INTUBATION

Early in his career the anaesthetist learns the value of being able to intubate patients during anaesthesia and becomes expert with this technique. It is, however, not only the anaesthetist who will find this a valuable manoeuvre, for intubation of the trachea is of value to the paediatrician, the obstetrician, the surgeon, the general practitioner and all doctors dealing with emergency cases. The full value of this procedure becomes apparent when one considers the indications for carrying it out.

Indications for Endotracheal Intubation

1. MAINTENANCE OF A CLEAR AIRWAY UNDER DIFFICULT CIRCUMSTANCES. In anaesthetic practice this usually means when the patient is lying on his side, on his face or when the head may have to be placed in an awkward position. On rare occasions it may be the only way of ensuring a clear airway even in the supine position in the unconscious patient who has a large tongue or in whom it is otherwise difficult to maintain the airway.

2. TO ALLOW PROPER CONTROL OF ANAESTHESIA DURING OPERATIONS ON THE HEAD, NECK, MOUTH, THROAT AND NOSE. This form of anaesthesia is used extensively in all operations around the head and neck where it would be impracticable to administer the anaesthetic through a facepiece or mask without interfering with surgical access.

3. TO PROTECT THE TRACHEA FROM CONTAMINATION. The use of a cuffed endotracheal tube will ensure that the anaesthetic can be delivered to the lungs and at the same time will prevent any material such as blood, mucus, pus or vomitus from gaining access to the trachea and also to the lungs. Anaesthesia is therefore maintained via a cuffed endotracheal tube in ear, nose and throat operations, dental and other oral

procedures and in patients liable to vomit or regurgitate during anaesthesia, for instance obstetric cases and cases of intestinal obstruction.

4. To Reduce the Anatomical Dead Space. Intubation may be used during anaesthesia where the introduction of an endotracheal tube will halve the anatomical dead space. It may also be employed in such cases as head injuries or in patients with respiratory insufficiency where again reduction of the dead space is a valuable contribution towards the resuscitation and management of these cases. This may be a temporary measure prior to tracheostomy (see Chapter XI).

5. To Facilitate Tracheo-bronchial Toilet. An endotracheal tube may be passed either during anaesthesia or in the post-operative phase to facilitate tracheo-bronchial suction through a catheter. While it is desirable when looking for a discrete blockage of a bronchus, such as by a plug of mucus, to pass a bronchoscope and to aspirate it under direct vision, it is often possible, where secretions are diffuse and widespread and no discrete plug is suspected, to aspirate more easily through an endotracheal tube. This causes less disturbance to the patient than does a bronchoscopy and it enables oxygenation of the apnoeic patient to be continued more adequately than during bronchoscopy.

6. As a Means of Facilitating Controlled Ventilation. It is desirable in cases where controlled ventilation is to be continued over a long period to intubate the trachea so that gases are not blown into the stomach causing gastric distension and possible regurgitation. It should be stressed that endotracheal intubation is not the first essential in resuscitation and that artificial ventilation can be started before intubating the trachea.

Therapeutic Indications for Endotracheal Intubation

Any patient who is likely to be unconscious for a period of more than 24 hours should have an endotracheal tube passed. This ensures a good airway and allows tracheo-bronchial toilet to be carried out at any time. Thus there are indications for endotracheal intubation in poisonings such as by barbiturate or coal gas, in head injuries and in cerebrovascular catastrophes.

In patients with post-operative respiratory insufficiency, the use of an endotracheal tube may reduce the dead space sufficiently to allow the patient to breathe adequately until some recovery of function takes place. Alternatively, this measure may be a temporary procedure before tracheostomy is considered.

In resuscitation of the new-born the passage of an endotracheal tube facilitates artificial ventilation and endobronchial suction to clear the air passages of mucus. In other forms of resuscitation, as in cardiac arrest or drowning, the ability to pass an endotracheal tube may also be invaluable.

In describing the technique of endotracheal intubation, we will consider briefly the induction of adequate anaesthesia for its performance but clearly in many conditions, such as in resuscitation and emergencies, no anaesthesia is necessary, desirable or even possible. The other considerations, however, are equally applicable both to anaesthesia and resuscitation.

There are three essentials for the successful passage of a tube into the trachea.

1. Adequate anaesthesia and relaxation of the muscles of the head, neck and larynx.
2. Proper positioning of the head and neck.
3. The use of the correct apparatus for the procedure.

Anaesthesia for Endotracheal Intubation

Endotracheal intubation during anaesthesia is only part of an anaesthetic technique and seldom an end in itself. Therefore the anaesthetist normally induces anaesthesia with a sleep dose of thiopentone and follows this with a full dose of muscle relaxant.

While local analgesia may be used to facilitate the introduction of an endotracheal tube where this is being done to allow endobronchial suction in cases with retained secretions post-operatively, care must always be taken to avoid toxic dosage of the local agents. Using the 4 per cent. solution of lignocaine it is easy to exceed the maximum dose of the drug.

Posture of Patients for Endotracheal Intubation

The classic description of the correct posture for endotracheal intubation is that the neck should be slightly flexed and the head extended. This has been described as the "sniffing the air position". It is illustrated correctly in Figure 53, from which it can be seen that with the head and neck in this

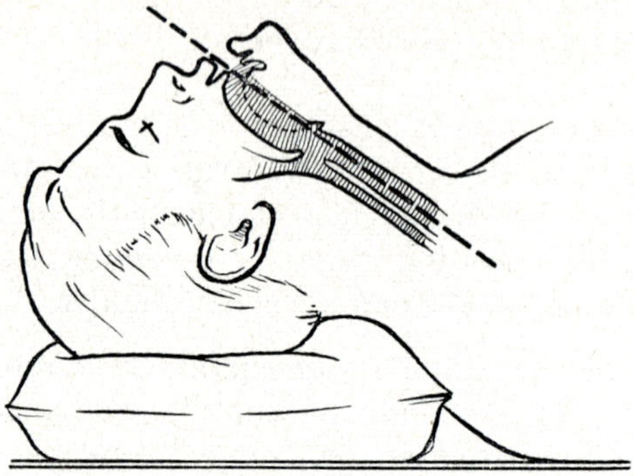

FIG. 53
The correct posture of head and neck for laryngoscopy. With the neck flexed and the head extended, the mouth, laryngoscope and trachea are in a straight line.

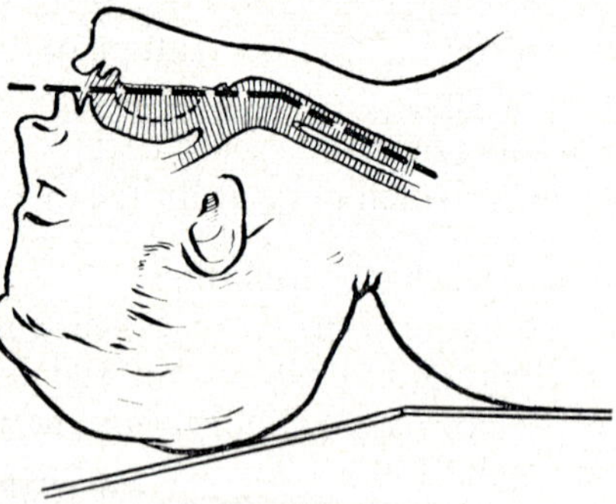

FIG. 54
The incorrect posture for laryngoscopy. With the neck extended and head extended, the trachea and laryngoscope blade are no longer in line.

position there is a straight line from the mouth through the vocal cords and down the trachea which of course has a 10° backward tilt. The common mistake is to extend the neck and the head. This position is shown in Figure 54 and the difficulties which arise from its use can be clearly seen. One is looking uphill to see the larynx while the trachea then runs downhill and in fact the tube has to be passed through quite a considerable angle. Appreciation of this relatively simple point can save a great deal of trouble during intubation.

Apparatus for Endotracheal Intubation

The apparatus to be considered is that for direct or blind intubation and consists of a variety of laryngoscopes, endotracheal tubes, aids to introduction of the endotracheal tube, sprays for producing local analgesia of the larynx and connectors to connect the endotracheal tubes to the anaesthetic apparatus or ventilator.

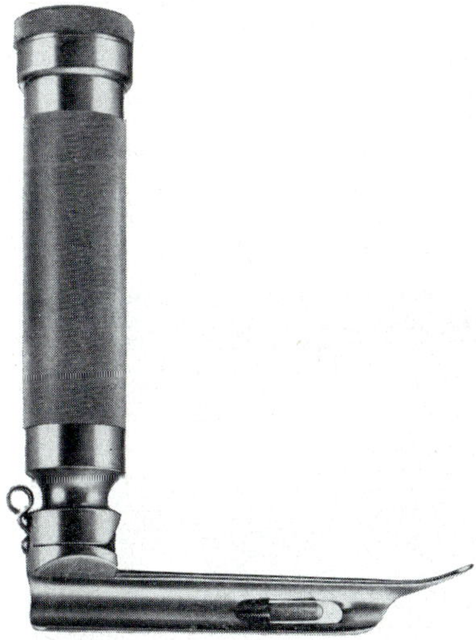

FIG. 55
The Magill laryngoscope.

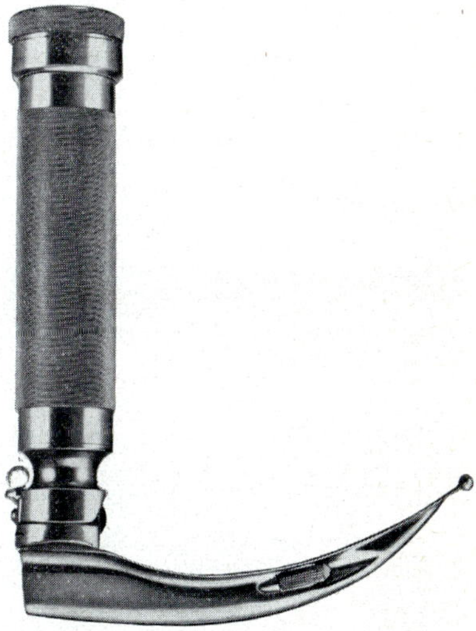

FIG. 56
The Macintosh laryngoscope.

LARYNGOSCOPES are divided into two groups, those with straight blades and those with curved blades. The first typified by the Magill laryngoscope shown in Figure 55 is passed over the base of tongue and posterior to the epiglottis exposing the larynx in a straight line. As the posterior surface of the epiglottis is supplied by the vagus nerve, reflexes set up by the use of this instrument tend to cause laryngeal spasm and a fairly deep level of anaesthesia is required. To avoid this difficulty, the Macintosh laryngoscope (Fig. 56) was designed to pass over the base of the tongue but into the vallecula anterior to the epiglottis, an area which is supplied by the glossopharyngeal nerve. Figures 57 and 58 show the two instruments in use, and illustrate this point. Although

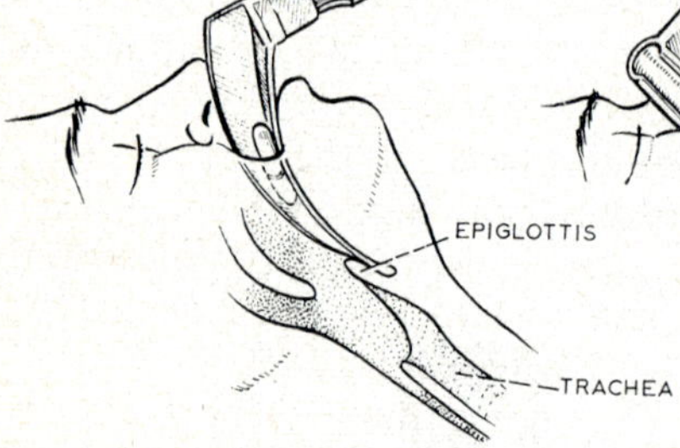

FIG. 57

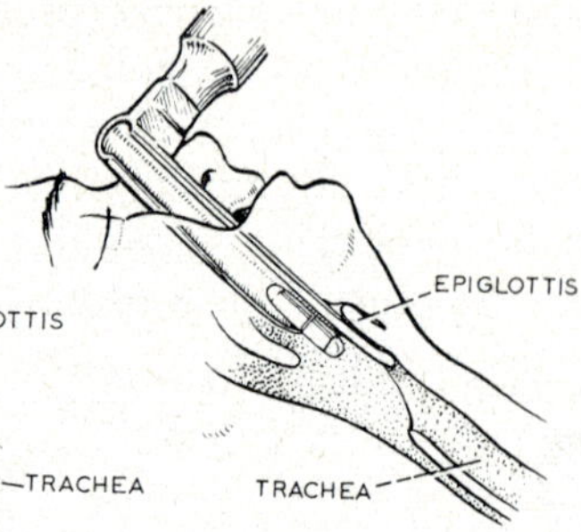

FIG. 58

Figure 57 shows the Macintosh laryngoscope in use. The blade tip is anterior to the epiglottis.

Figure 58 shows the Magill laryngoscope in use. The blade tip is posterior to the epiglottis.

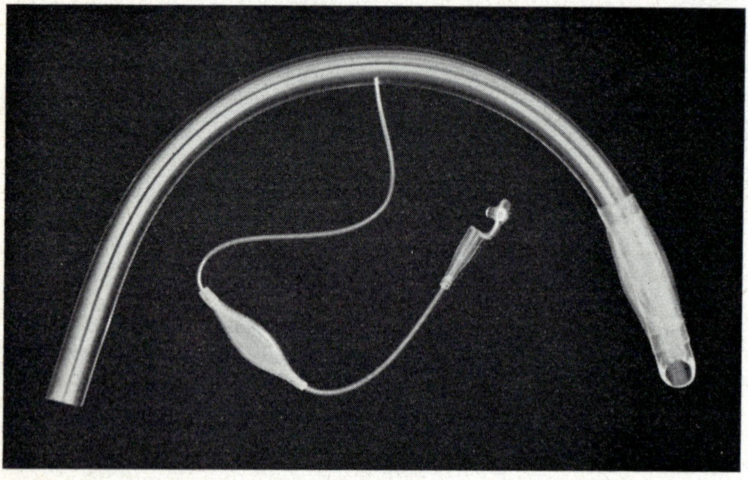

FIG. 59
A cuffed " Portex " tube.

with the introduction of muscle relaxants and the widespread use of these drugs for intubation the original indications for the Macintosh laryngoscope have perhaps disappeared, these instruments are very widely used nowadays and with a few exceptions are universally applicable.

ENDOTRACHEAL TUBES vary considerably in design. The plain endotracheal tube for use in the mouth or nose and the cuffed endotracheal tubes for use through the mouth are illustrated in Figures 59 and 60. A tube of appropriate size chosen from one of these three types will satisfy most needs. Thus

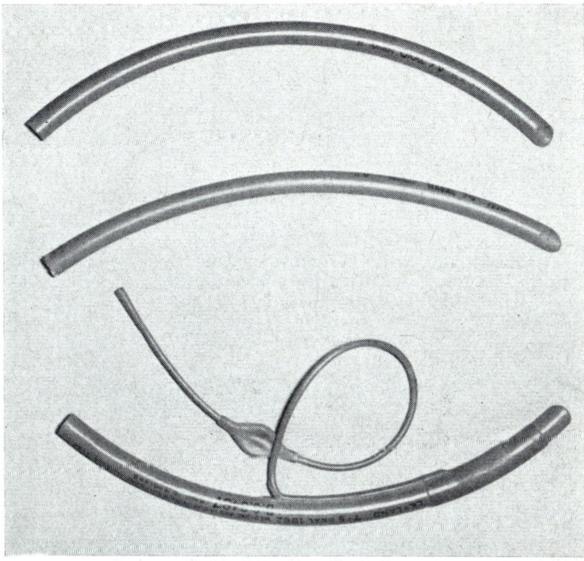

FIG. 60
Three types of rubber endotracheal tubes in common use: from above down, plain, oral and nasal tubes and a cuffed oral tube.

a cuffed tube will provide a clear airway and protect the trachea from soiling. In small children or in patients where the use of a cuff is considered undesirable a plain oral tube may be used along with a mouth pack. Oral operations or dental procedures may be performed using a nasal endotracheal tube. These tubes are made of thinner material so that the internal diameter is slightly larger than the oral equivalent.

In certain circumstances when the head is to be put into an extremely difficult position such as in some forms of neurosurgery or where a gag has to be placed in the mouth over the tube as during cleft palate or hare lip surgery or during tonsillectomy, some reinforcement of the side of the tube may be required to prevent it kinking or being compressed. Various forms of reinforced tubes are available. In some cases a rubber tube is reinforced with a metal spiral or a latex tube may be used where again a metal spiral is embedded in the wall of the tube. Another tube less commonly used is formed by fusing

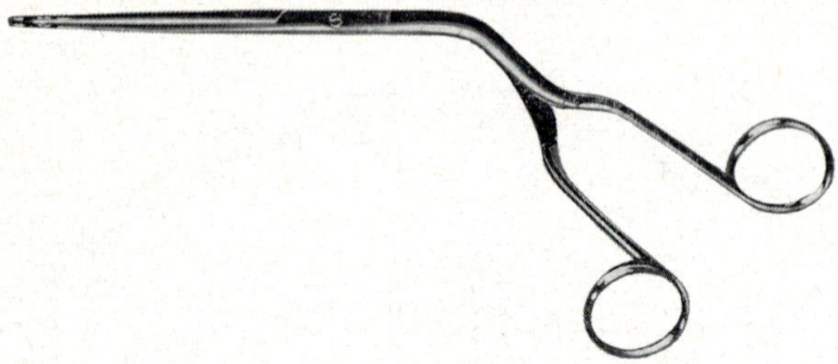

FIG. 61
The Magill intubating forceps, curved to allow their use in the mouth, are used to guide an endotracheal tube through the vocal cords.

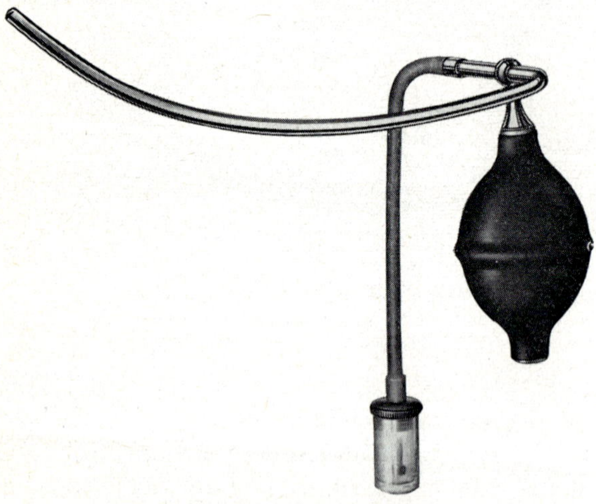

FIG. 62
The Forrester laryngeal spray. The container for the analgesic has a maximum capacity of 4 ml. The metal part of the spray fits the curvature of a Macintosh laryngoscope.

over the upper portion of a plain endotracheal tube a larger tube, so that the part which goes into the larynx is of the size appropriate to the patient while the upper portion of the tube is in fact of double the thickness. Many other modifications of the plain endotracheal tube have been described.

INTUBATING FORCEPS (Fig. 61) may be used to pick up the tip of an endotracheal tube and introduce it through the cords where the anatomy of the mouth is such that it would otherwise be deflected into the oesophagus.

LARYNGEAL SPRAYS have been designed to facilitate the deposition of a fine mist of local analgesic solution on the cords, the piriform fossae and through the cords into the trachea. This is desirable even when general anaesthesia is employed so that reflexes caused by the tube as it passes through the cords into the trachea may be minimised. One such spray is shown in Figure 62.

CONNECTORS designed to join the endotracheal tube to the anaesthetic apparatus are shown in Figure 63. The choice of

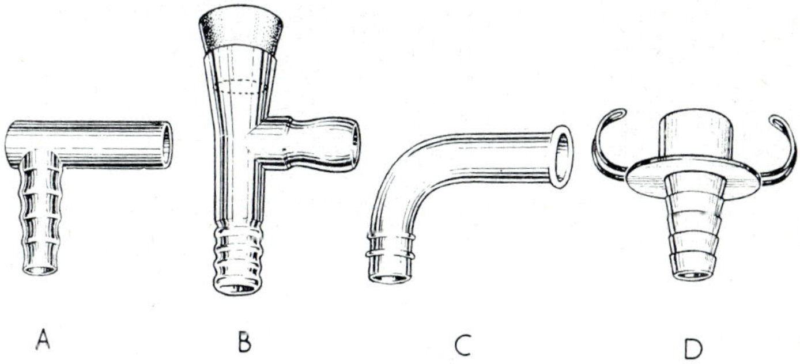

FIG. 63 A-D
Endotracheal tube connectors.

A. The Rowbotham connector. The right angle causes turbulent flow which increases resistance during respiration.
B. A suction connector. The rubber cork can be removed to allow the passage of a suction catheter without disconnecting the tube.
C. A curved connector which reduces turbulence and thus the resistance to respiration.
D. The Forrester connector. This connector is straight and of wide bore. Resistance to respiration is minimal and endotracheal suction is easily performed.

connector depends on many factors. If surgical access to the face or nose is of prime importance then a Magill or Rowbotham connector will be chosen (Fig. 63C and A). If, however, aspiration of the trachea during operation is contemplated a suction connector such as shown at Figure 63B is preferable. For general use we find the Forrester connector (Fig 63D) to be almost ideal. It does not require a catheter mount to join it to the anaesthetic machine or bellows and it fits directly to the angle piece and the expiratory valve. This, apart from its obvious simplicity, allows a wide bore tube to be used throughout and reduces the resistance to respiration.

More recently plastic connectors have become available, one of which is shown at Figure 63 E.

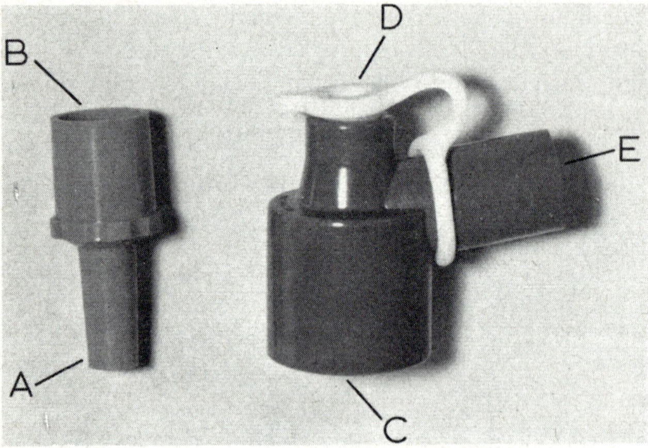

FIG. 63 E. The Portex endotracheal connector and swivel mount. This may be used as a unit by connecting A to the endotracheal tube, B to C and E to a catheter mount and thus to the anaesthetic machine. In this case, suction catheters may be passed into the trachea by lifting the cap D. Alternatively, using the modern British Standard connector, B may be joined directly to the delivery tube from the machine.

In addition to choosing an appropriate connector for the operation to be carried out, it is important to use one of the largest diameter that will fit easily into the endotracheal tube. This is important because the effective diameter of a series of tubes is the smallest diameter of the series. It is useless to pass a large endotracheal tube and join it to a narrow connector.

The Technique of Endotracheal Intubation

Before taking any steps towards intubating the trachea, it is important that everything should be at hand so that there is no delay once the procedure has started. The chosen laryngoscope should be tested and laid close at hand and intubating forceps, spray and connector should be easily available. In selecting a tube the anaesthetist will decide whether a cuffed tube is to be employed or whether a plain tube is to be passed through the mouth or through the nose and a selection of suitable sizes will be available. Until recently the numbers on the endotracheal tube have indicated the size of the tubes, ranging from the "00" tube to be used in neonates to the number 12 tube used for the largest adults. More recently, however, the size of the tube is given in mm. (Fig. 64).

Magill Number	Mm. Internal Diameter	
	Oral	Nasal
00	3·0	
0A	3·5	
0	4·0	
1	4·5	
2	5·0	5·5
3	5·5	6·0
4	6·0	6·5
5	6·5	7·0
6	7·0	7·5
7	7·5	8·0
8	8·0	8·5
9	9·0	9·0
10	9·5	10·0
11	10·0	
12	11·0	

FIG. 64

The selection of the appropriate bore of tube is based roughly on the patient's age. In this way the patient's age plus one may be taken and this figure halved to give a rough indication of the Magill number of tube required. Thus a child of seven will normally take a Magill number 4 endotracheal tube. Alternatively by dividing the child's age by 4 and adding 4·5 the size in mm. may be estimated. Since there is however a considerable variation in the size of the larynx in different patients, it is usual to use this only as a rough guide to the size probably required and to lay out a tube larger and smaller than the one selected by this rule. For adults, a female will usually require a 9 or 9·5 mm. tube, a male 9·5 to 11 mm. tube.

A rough guide to the *correct length* of tube required can be obtained by measuring the distance from the lobe of the ear to the angle of the mouth, for oral intubation, or the nose for nasal intubation. A tube cut to twice this length should reach from the incisor teeth or nostril to the mid-point of the trachea.

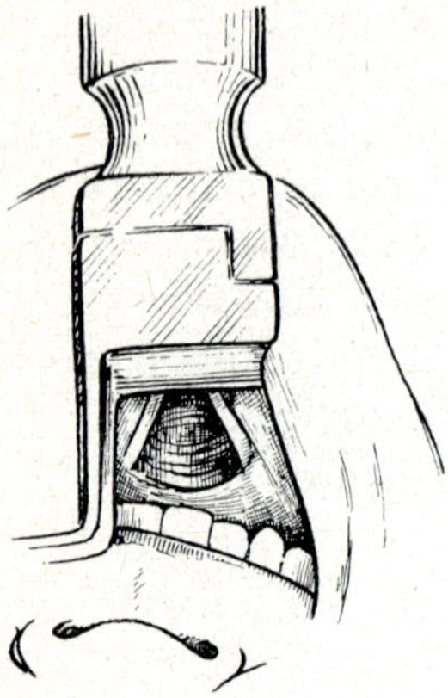

FIG. 65
The view of the larynx and trachea obtained on direct laryngoscopy.

The laryngoscope is introduced into the patient's mouth and the tip of the laryngoscope is then slipped over the tongue until the epiglottis comes into sight. At this point, if a Magill laryngoscope is being used, the epiglottis is lifted forward, whereas if a Macintosh laryngoscope is used, the tip of the laryngoscope is inserted into the vallecula and the base of the tongue lifted forward, carrying the epiglottis with it.

A view such as shown in Figure 65 will then be obtained.

At this stage if there is no danger of inhalation of vomitus or blood at the end of operation, one may decide to spray the vocal cords and through the cords into the trachea with a local analgesic. If so a suitable local analgesic spray is used and a small dose, normally not more than 4 ml. of 4 per cent. lignocaine, is sprayed in the area. Similarly where there is no danger from inhalation after extubation, a local analgesic lubricant is applied to the tube before intubating the trachea. In cases of intestinal obstruction or in operations on the mouth, throat or nose where blood may be present in the pharynx at the end of operation, a non-analgesic lubricant such as " KY " jelly is preferred.

Having passed a cuffed tube, one must inflate the cuff by means of the side tube or insert a pharyngeal pack and connect the tube to the anaesthetic apparatus. The anaesthetic is then continued using any selected method.

When inflating the cuff on the tube it is important to remember that the small pilot balloon at the end of the cuff merely indicates when there is air in the tube and cuff. The degree of distension of the pilot balloon gives no guide to the degree of distension of the cuff on the endotracheal tube itself as this depends on their relative elasticity.

After the endotracheal tube has been placed in position it is sometimes very difficult to ventilate the patient and this is often due to kinking of the tube. This diagnosis can be confirmed by passing a finger into the mouth and feeling the kink where it occurs. It may be abolished by correct positioning of the head and sometimes the introduction of an airway into the mouth will also help to reduce the incidence of this complication. Where kinking persists or recurs and the tube is liable to be in position for a long time it is advisable to remove the tube and insert a stronger one. Occasionally the tube may pass into the right bronchus causing collapse of the left lung (see p. 268).

Complications of Endotracheal Intubation

The complications of intubation are divided into the minor fairly common and troublesome ones such as sore throat and damage to the pharynx, and serious ones which are relatively uncommon such as laryngeal oedema and granuloma.

Sore throat is common following endotracheal anaesthesia and probably is found in about 50 per cent. of all patients. The incidence may be reduced by extreme care during the introduction of the tube and also by its adequate sterilisation as minor infection is probably a contributory factor. Adequate lubrication of the endotracheal tube will tend to reduce the incidence of sore throat and avoidance of throat packs will also help, though sometimes a carefully placed throat pack by stopping movement of the tube during the anaesthetic assists in reduction of this complication. Treatment consists largely of mild analgesics, mouth washes and perhaps inhalations of Tinct. Benz. Co. vapour.

Oedema of the larynx leads to laryngeal stridor and partial or complete obstruction of the airway. It is often associated with the use of too large an endotracheal tube or excessive force being used to pass the tube through the larynx. It is most commonly found in children and those with a small airway. The onset of stridor after endotracheal anaesthesia heralds the occurrence of laryngeal oedema and inhalation of humidified oxygen and Tinct. Benz. Co. or menthol vapour may help to reduce its severity. In severe cases helium may be added to the oxygen to facilitate its inhalation into the trachea or bronchi and a tracheostomy may be required as a temporary measure to alleviate an obstruction due to oedema. An antibiotic is useful to combat infection. Laryngeal granulomata are the province of the ear, nose and throat surgeon and are an unusual complication of endotracheal intubation and bronchoscopy.

SPECIAL TUBES AND BLOCKERS

While we have described tubes suitable for endotracheal anaesthesia and these are normally passed to a point midway between the cords and the bifurcation of the trachea, there are others designed particularly for thoracic operations. Such tubes are longer and are passed into one or other main bronchus so that the anaesthetic may be maintained via one lung while the other is allowed to collapse during the operation. These endobronchial tubes are narrower in diameter than the endotracheal ones and have a small cuff so that it will not obstruct the other bronchi once placed in the main stem bronchus.

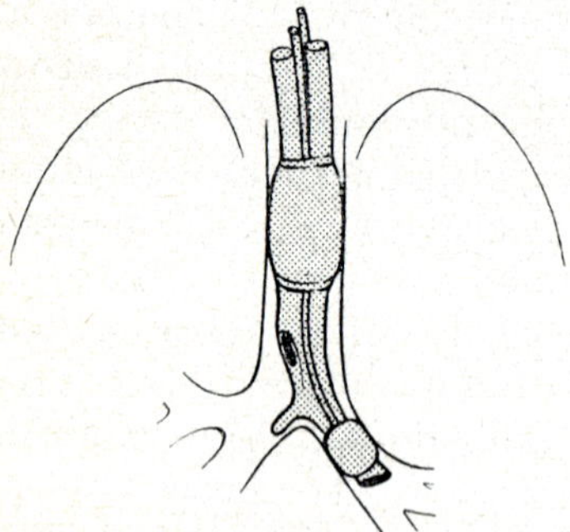

FIG. 66
The Carlens double lumen tube. One or other lung can be ventilated independently.

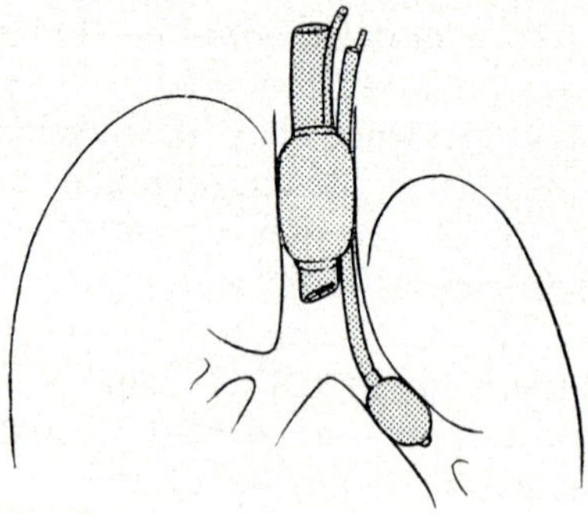

FIG. 67
A bronchus blocker in position alongside an endotracheal tube. The left lung is partially collapsed by suction through the blocker.

The administration of an anaesthetic into one lung is of particular value where the other lung is to be removed and there are occasions when the anaesthetist may wish to inflate the lungs independently of one another. For this purpose double lumen tubes, as for example the Carlens' tube (Fig. 66), or Robertshaw's tube may be used.

An alternative technique used where only part of the lung is to be removed and particularly where there are profuse secretions from the diseased lobe, is to pass a long suction catheter with a cuff at the end into the bronchus supplying the diseased lobe. Such a catheter, known as a bronchus blocker, is shown in Figure 67. This blocker is passed through a bronchoscope and accurately positioned and thereafter the anaesthetic is maintained via an endotracheal tube.

BRONCHOSCOPY

Bronchoscopy, once the province of the ear, nose and throat surgeon, is now a technique employed by many other practitioners. The thoracic surgeon frequently uses the bronchoscope, the physician similarly may employ bronchoscopy and the anaesthetist is also expected to be able to use such an instrument.

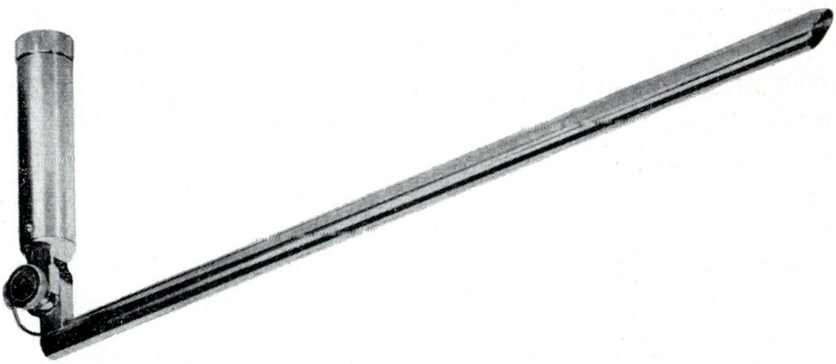

FIG. 68
A bronchoscope with battery in the handle suitable for emergency use.

The indications for bronchoscopy, in anaesthetic practice, are the removal of secretions from the tracheo-bronchial tree post-operatively and the removal of foreign bodies from the lungs. One may use a bronchoscope as illustrated in Figure 68 with the battery stored in the handle. The technique is particularly applicable to the removal of discrete plugs blocking a bronchus or to the exploration of the left lung where suction through an endotracheal tube is less liable to be successful because of the more acute angle of the left bronchus.

The initial position of the patient's head for bronchoscopy is the same as for laryngoscopy but thereafter the position of the head must be altered so that the bronchoscope passes readily down the trachea and then enters the bronchus in correct alignment. This involves considerable repositioning of the head and the help of an assistant should be available.

The anaesthetic technique for bronchoscopy varies considerably. Local analgesic preparation may be employed without rendering the patient unconscious. A general anaesthetic may be used, inducing anaesthesia to a deep level with a non-inflammable anaesthetic such as halothane and allowing the patient to breathe spontaneously throughout. This technique is however not very popular. An alternative is to induce anaesthesia with thiopentone and a short-acting relaxant such as suxamethonium, to spray the vocal cords and trachea with a local analgesic and then introduce the bronchoscope. Thereafter the patient is allowed to breathe spontaneously and the local analgesic prevents bucking and coughing during the procedure.

Maintenance of ventilation during bronchoscopy is however difficult although many bronchoscopes are equipped with a side tube which carries the gas to the lungs. Alternatively a small catheter may be passed alongside the bronchoscope. This allows oxygen and a volatile agent to be insufflated during bronchoscopy and is a reasonable compromise.

For further details the reader is referred to the excellent work by Noel Gillespie on endotracheal anaesthesia.

CHAPTER IX

THE PREVENTION AND TREATMENT OF COMPLICATIONS DURING ANAESTHESIA

In addition to watching for signs that the level of anaesthesia is adequate for the operation in hand, one must prevent certain complications or treat them if and when they occur. Some of these complications are common unless steps are routinely taken to prevent them, whereas others are unusual and unexpected hazards. Many, such as vomiting, may occur at any time during anaesthesia or the recovery period but some are associated more often with one phase of the anaesthetic. Where a complication is discussed in more than one section, stress is laid on the measures used in prevention and treatment at that stage of the anaesthetic.

COMPLICATIONS AND DIFFICULTIES DURING INDUCTION OF ANAESTHESIA

Intravenous induction of anaesthesia may be complicated by:

1. The Injection of Thiopentone, in Error, into an Artery when severe vasospasm will result and damage to the intima may be followed by thrombosis. Although this danger can be minimised by routine use of 2·5 per cent. thiopentone and by avoiding the sites where arteries are known to lie in close proximity to the intended vein, it is advisable that one should know how to deal with this complication. When the patient complains of severe pain during injection it is always tempting immediately to withdraw the needle from the vein but this temptation should be resisted. Instead, through the needle one may inject 1 per cent. procaine, which will help to dilate the vessel and to reduce the pain of the previous thiopentone injection. Measures directed to relieve the vasospasm have been used such as the injection of tolazoline (Priscol) 5 ml. of 1 per cent. solution intra-arterially and stellate ganglion block. However, it has been shown that the vasoconstriction is very transient and these measures are considered less important than hitherto.

The main danger arises from the thrombosis which takes place in the vessel due to the intimal damage. This can be avoided or minimised by the prompt administration of an adequate dose of heparin to the patient (3 mg./Kg.). Where possible operation should be postponed and anticoagulant therapy continued for some days. If, however, this is not possible the heparin may still be administered and neutralised with the appropriate dose of protamine at the end of the operation. As this regime will clearly add considerable risk to any operation the importance placed on prophylaxis, that is avoiding sites where arteries may be entered and the use of a 2·5 per cent. solution, cannot be over-emphasised (see also p. 260).

Methohexitone 1 per cent. and propanidid are safer than thiopentone 2·5 per cent. in this respect.

2. PERIVENOUS INJECTION OF THE DRUG. This is seldom serious if the anaesthetist is vigilant. The administration of as little as 1 or 2 ml. of solution outside the vein will cause pain and will show as a small bleb or swelling at the point of the needle. If the injection is discontinued at this stage, little harm will probably be done but it is usual to inject into the area where the perivenous injection has taken place a solution containing 1 per cent. procaine and hyaluronidase (up to 10 ml. with 1,000 I.U. hyaluronidase). This deals with the situation in three ways.

(*i*) It reduces the pain.

(*ii*) It causes vasodilatation.

(*iii*) It dilutes the solution of thiopentone and spreads it over a wider area. The latter two factors enable the thiopentone to be absorbed from the tissues before any damage is done.

3. COUGHING, BREATH HOLDING AND LARYNGEAL SPASM are often encountered during induction of anaesthesia by inhalational means where an attempt is being made to introduce irritant vapours too rapidly. Normally a temporary reduction in concentration of the agent with, perhaps, the administration of a little carbon dioxide will deal with the patient who is coughing or holding his breath. A mild laryngeal stridor may respond similarly but the treatment of severe laryngeal spasm is more rigorous (p. 128).

4. AIRWAY OBSTRUCTION must be avoided throughout induction of anaesthesia and this is normally achieved by holding

forward the chin so that the tongue is kept clear of the pharynx. Unless it is absolutely essential an artificial airway should not be inserted during induction of anaesthesia, as, when the patient is lightly anaesthetised, this often causes retching and vomiting. If an airway must be inserted it should be well lubricated with an analgesic paste and preferably only partially inserted lest the tip go too far and cause a laryngeal spasm.

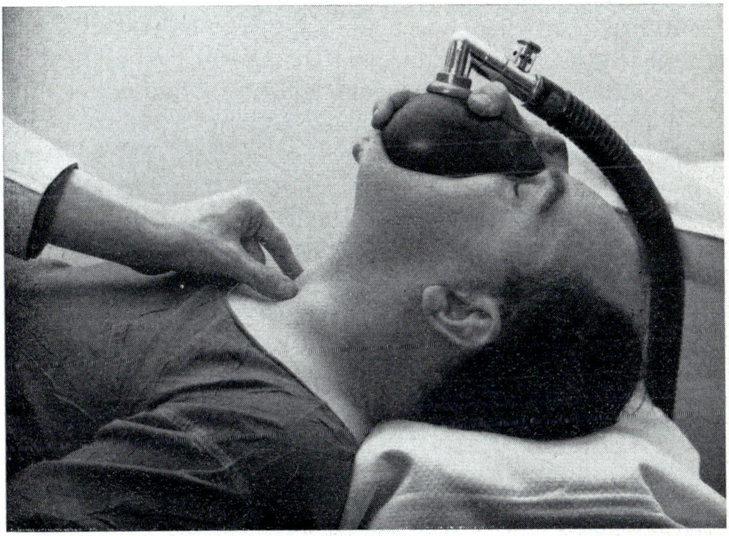

FIG. 69
Pressure on the cricoid by an assistant, during induction of anaesthesia, may prevent regurgitation of stomach contents.

In addition to the desirability of allowing free passage of the anaesthetic agents into the lungs, the airway must be kept clear for other reasons also. Where obstruction takes place and respiratory effort is continuing, a negative pressure is induced in the pharynx which leads to incompetence of the cardiac sphincter and regurgitation of stomach content may take place.

5. VOMITING or regurgitation during induction of anaesthesia is a hazardous complication. In addition to taking all the appropriate precautions *before* induction of anaesthesia, pressure on the cricoid cartilage (Fig. 69) during induction of anaesthesia may compress the oesophagus and reduce the likeli-

hood of regurgitation of gastric contents until a cuffed endotracheal tube can be passed.

If vomiting or regurgitation does occur the only safe way of dealing with it is to discontinue the induction, turn the patient on to his side with his head low and clear the pharynx by suction or swabbing. When this has been done, induction of anaesthesia must be continued as quickly as possible, preferably with the patient on his side and still with his head low. This is not as difficult as it sounds. When anaesthesia has been induced with inhalational agents from the start, it is probable that the patient has retained his laryngeal reflexes and will cough out any vomitus and thus will not inhale any. If induction has been achieved by the use of thiopentone, the severe laryngeal spasm will probably similarly protect the tracheobronchial tree and only if a muscle relaxant has been given or the patient is feeble or frail is there any real likelihood of inhalation of stomach content during induction. If this does occur, however, it is a serious complication and the operation should probably be postponed if possible while it is dealt with. The treatment is discussed at a later stage (p. 141).

COMPLICATIONS DURING MAINTENANCE OF ANAESTHESIA

The complications may be considered in three groups.

RESPIRATORY COMPLICATIONS

During anaesthesia with spontaneous respiration, the reservoir bag may either cease to move or do so with diminished amplitude. There are two possible causes for this.

1. Respiration may have been depressed even to the point of apnoea.

2. Respiration may be obstructed, partially or completely.

It is extremely important to differentiate between these two groups as the treatment is entirely different. This is, however, not difficult. When the patient is apnoeic no movement takes place in the reservoir bag and no respiratory effort is observed in the patient. On the other hand, when respiration is obstructed, there is diminished or absent movement in the reservoir bag but exaggerated respiratory effort is present. Noisy respiration is often associated with obstruction of the airway.

The distinction between the two groups is extremely important because respiratory depression or apnoea can be adequately treated in the first instance, by assisting or controlling ventilation with a mixture containing at least atmospheric proportions of oxygen and specific treatment can be carried out later when the exact cause of the depression is established. On the other hand, before respiratory obstruction can be adequately treated, the cause must be known, since widely differing measures may be indicated. The treatment appropriate for one cause of obstruction is not only useless for others, but may, indeed, make them worse.

Respiratory Depression

Respiratory depression may be central or peripheral. Central causes include the use of heavy doses of narcotics in premedication, the administration of excessive doses of thiopentone, or large doses of potent anaesthetic agents such as ether or halothane. If respiration has been assisted for a short time, lowered tension of carbon dioxide in the blood may also be a contributory factor.

Peripheral causes include any measures which have blocked the myoneural junction and may include the specific muscle relaxants. The regional techniques such as spinal or epidural block and potent anaesthetic agents such as ether also act peripherally.

During anaesthesia, the anaesthetist will normally assist ventilation if it is inadequate and if he suspects that a volatile agent is responsible for the respiratory depression, will reduce the concentration. While specific antagonists may be used to overcome the depression produced by thiopentone, narcotic or indeed by muscle relaxant drugs it is unusual to administer these in the course of an anaesthetic but rather to assist ventilation until the end of anaesthesia.

Respiratory Obstruction

Respiratory obstruction may also arise from a variety of causes. It is convenient to consider these from the anaesthetic machine to the respiratory tract starting at the lips and finishing in the alveoli.

1. The Anaesthetic Machine and Apparatus. It is unusual for the delivery tubes on the anaesthetic machines to kink or become blocked, as they are specifically designed to avoid this but very unusual positions or pressure on the tube may obstruct the flow of gases to the patient. In addition, if rebreathing is taking place into the tubing, moisture from the exhalations may condense in the expiratory limb and water

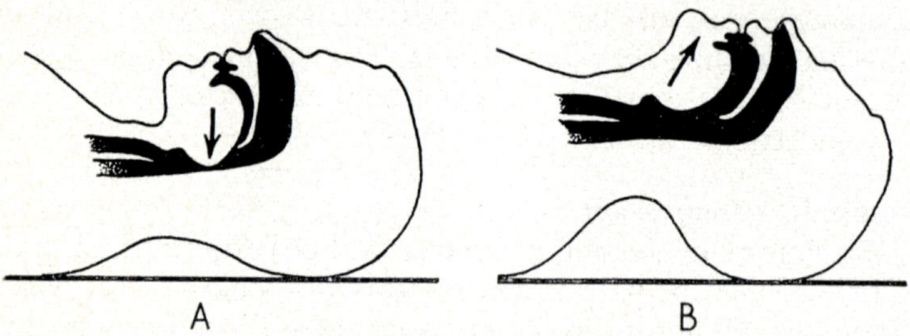

Fig. 70

These figures demonstrate the correct positioning of the head and jaw during anaesthesia and mouth-to-mouth breathing to ensure a clear airway. In A the head is slightly flexed, the jaw is unsupported and the tongue has fallen back obstructing the upper airway. In B the head has been extended, the jaw pulled forward taking the tongue with it and clearing the airway.

in dependent parts may cause a partial obstruction. The other common cause of respiratory obstruction in anaesthetic apparatus is an endotracheal tube kinking during anaesthesia. This possibility is considered further in the section on endotracheal intubation (p. 117).

2. The Lips may cause obstruction, particularly in edentulous patients. When the chin is supported, the lips may not only obstruct the mouth but may also press on the nares, obstructing respiration through the nose. This complication is treated by insertion of a small lubricated oral airway.

3. The Tongue. This is one of the commonest causes of obstruction of the airway during anaesthesia. During anaesthesia and indeed during normal sleep the muscles around the jaw relax and the mandible falls backward carrying with it the tongue which is attached to it. This is shown in Figure 70. As a result, the tongue falls backwards and makes contact with the

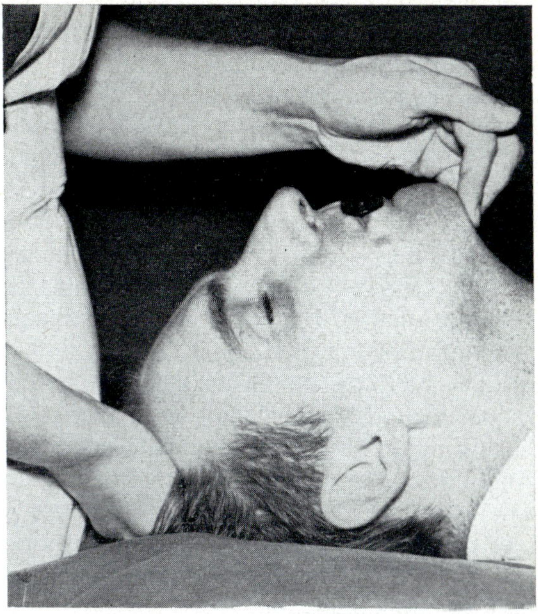

FIG. 71

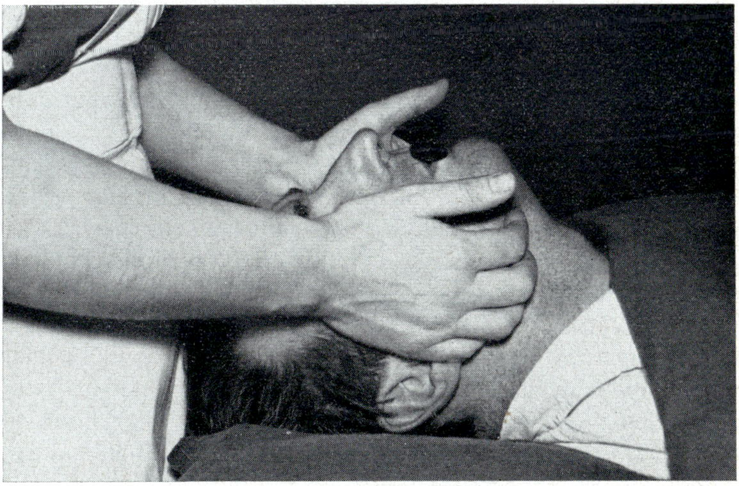

FIG. 72

FIGS. 71 and 72. Two alternative methods of supporting the unconscious patient's chin to prevent upper airway obstruction. Whether the tip of the chin or the angles of the jaw are supported the direction of the pull is the same.

posterior pharyngeal wall, completely obstructing the oropharynx. This may result in a noise similar to snoring. It is treated by supporting the mandible as shown in Figures 71 and 72 or again by insertion of an airway. When inserting an airway in the lightly anaesthetised patient care must again be taken not to push it too far back and to lubricate it adequately.

4. THE PHARYNX may be occluded by vomitus, false teeth or blood. In this case the treatment is to lower the head and clear the obstruction by suction or other appropriate means.

5. DISEASE PROCESSES around the larynx are rare causes of respiratory obstruction. Epiglottic cysts and tumours of the vocal cords are examples of such.

6. LARYNGEAL STRIDOR OR SPASM are common causes of respiratory obstruction during light anaesthesia. Laryngeal stridor, which is caused by an incomplete closure of the vocal cords during inspiration, is detected by the presence of a characteristic high pitched sound during inspiration. Laryngeal spasm where the cords are completely closed is noiseless but, in both cases, the obstruction to respiration is accompanied by exaggerated respiratory effort.

Stridor or spasm may arise from two distinct sets of causes. In the first place, local irritation of the cords by inhalation of irritant vapours such as ether, by fluids such as vomitus or by solid bodies such as an artificial airway may all cause laryngeal spasm. This is a protective measure designed to prevent contamination of the tracheo-bronchial tree.

Stridor and spasm may also occur reflexly, that is from impulses set up distant from the larynx itself as by incision of the skin, stretching of sphincters such as the anal sphincter, dilatation of the vagina or cervix and pulling on the peritoneum.

It is claimed by some that laryngeal stridor or spasm can be caused specifically by thiopentone. However, it seems more likely that while thiopentone depresses sympathetic more than parasympathetic activity, producing a state of relative parasympathetic over-activity, the actual cause of the spasm is probably irritation by nasopharyngeal mucus which is frequently present.

This complication results in partial or complete respiratory obstruction and the patient rapidly becomes hypoxic and retains carbon dioxide. It is claimed that in healthy patients the laryngeal stridor or spasm will always break before death takes place because, as the patient becomes grossly hypoxic, the laryngeal muscles finally weaken and the larynx relaxes to allow oxygen to pass before death occurs. This, of course, does not apply in patients who are already gravely ill and the anaesthetist should never risk seeing whether this sequence of events takes place.

Treatment is directed to removing the cause where this can be ascertained. Thus if a high concentration of ether is being administered this is reduced. If an airway has just been inserted, it should be partially withdrawn and, if it is suspected that fluid or vomitus is present in the pharynx, the head should be lowered and suction applied to the pharynx. Similarly, if the spasm occurs as the operation starts or as one of the manoeuvres described is taking place, surgical activity should cease temporarily.

If the spasm is only partial, that is if stridor is present, a high concentration of oxygen should be administered and when the spasm relaxes an attempt made to deepen anaesthesia so that it will not recur when the stimulus is re-applied. If spasm is complete, gentle pressure on the reservoir bag, which should be full of oxygen, is made in the hope that as the cords momentarily relax some oxygen will pass into the trachea. It is, of course, essential during these manoeuvres to ensure that the airway above the larynx is clear. If the spasm does not respond to such measures the anaesthetist would normally administer a small dose of a short acting relaxant, such as suxamethonium 50 mg., intravenously. This will produce complete muscle paralysis and ensure that the cords relax. When this has taken place, further attempts are made to deepen the anaesthetic so that the spasm will not recur when the muscle relaxant has worn off.

If a muscle relaxant is not available, other measures which have been described are to insert a needle through the cricothyroid membrane and spray local analgesic (such as 2-3 ml. lignocaine 4 per cent.) on the lower surface of the vocal cords. In addition, oxygen can be blown through a wide bore needle into the trachea as a temporary measure. Care must be taken to avoid building up a high pressure in the tracheo-bronchial tree in this way. This measure and the last resort, namely tracheostomy, should seldom be required.

7. OBSTRUCTION OF THE TRACHEA OR LARGE BRONCHI BY FOREIGN BODIES, such as vomitus, are possible but unusual causes of respiratory obstruction.

8. BRONCHOSPASM is a cause of respiratory obstruction which may be seen under certain circumstances. It is associated with the use of barbiturates and consequent relative parasympathetic over-activity. It is most common in patients who already have certain conditions in which bronchospasm is a feature, namely asthma and bronchitis. Where an endotracheal tube is in place the stimuli which have been noted as producing laryngeal spasm will often result instead in bronchospasm. Intense bronchospasm also accompanies the inhalation of acid gastric contents and is known as Mendelson's syndrome or the " acid aspiration syndrome ". This is characterised by severe bronchospasm, pulmonary oedema and circulatory failure. It is treated by administration of oxygen and hydrocortisone and is not normally an indication for bronchoscopy or for tracheobronchial suction, as the patients are often severely hypoxic and acid, which has caused the damage, is beyond the reach of a suction catheter. (See also p. 141.)

Bronchospasm, not associated with the inhalation of acid stomach content, may respond to measures designed to relax the bronchi, e.g. (*a*) aminophylline 250 mg. may be administered intravenously, (*b*) isoprenaline up to 1 ml. of 1 per cent. solution may be administered by a nebuliser. This drug is being superseded by orciprenaline, 0·5 mg. in 1 ml. intra-muscularly or 5-10 inhalations of aerosol solution (5-10 × 750 μg.), as it is longer acting and less liable to produce dangerous arrhythmias or by salbutamol which is claimed to have no cardiac side effects, (*c*) ether may be added to the anaesthetic mixture, (*d*) high concentrations of oxygen may be administered by positive pressure.

Inadequate Respiration

The above are some of the more dramatic complications which may be looked for, prevented, or treated during the maintenance of anaesthesia. However, of no less importance is the recognition of the less dramatic occurrence of inadequate respiration during the course of the anaesthetic. This is not the acute apnoea which is easily recognised and equally easily treated, but diminished respiratory volume, which leads to the accumulation of carbon dioxide and the slow development of hypoxia. Normally, when respiration is depressed during anaesthesia, both these states will occur. However, it is possible, in some circumstances, for hypoxia to occur without gross carbon dioxide retention and for carbon dioxide retention to occur without hypoxia.

Hypoxia without carbon dioxide retention may occur when a low inspired oxygen tension is administered. Such conditions are seen during nitrous oxide and oxygen anaesthesia, where no volatile supplement is used and a concentration of less than 33 per cent. oxygen is given. Similar conditions apply in non-anaesthetic circumstances where individuals are breathing at a high altitude, as when climbing mountains or when in a non-pressurised aircraft.

Similarly, carbon dioxide may be retained without obvious signs of hypoxia where a high concentration of oxygen is given. This occurs in anaesthetic practice where oxygen is used as the sole gas in administering oxygen and halothane anaesthesia. Halothane is a powerful respiratory depressant, if high concentrations are given, but the use of 100 per cent. oxygen to vaporise the drug masks the development of respiratory inadequacy by eliminating cyanosis. Similar considerations apply when giving cyclopropane with high concentrations of oxygen.

It should be noted that hypercarbia without hypoxia may also occur in a patient poisoned with barbiturates or in respiratory failure in a chronic bronchitic. The doctor admitting such a patient notices the cyanosis immediately, administers oxygen and, as the hypoxic drive is removed, the patient's respiration is depressed further and carbon dioxide accumulates in even higher concentrations.

Inadequate respiration may be detected in one of three ways:—

1. Direct measurements of the arterial blood gas levels may be made by determining the pH, Pa_{CO_2} and standard bicarbonate levels and the oxygen saturation and tension. Alternatively, the oxygen saturation may be determined by

using an oximeter. These techniques are not used in clinical anaesthetic practice as a routine but are employed during major surgery or where long term ventilation is being carried out.

2. An alternative method is to make external measurements of the respiratory minute volume. This may be done by using an instrument such as the Wright respirometer (Fig. 28). In this case the patient's basal requirements are calculated prior to anaesthesia from tables, such as the Radford nomogram, and the level of ventilation during anaesthesia maintained at this predicted value, using the respirometer as a constant check. Alternatively, it is possible to use the instrument to ensure that a minimum minute volume of 8 litres/minute is achieved by the patient either through his own efforts or with assistance from the anaesthetist. In this connection it is important to remember that allowance must be made for the dead space and that it is the *alveolar* minute volume which matters. The relationship of alveolar ventilation to Pa_{CO_2} is shown in Figure 73. A third method, where spontaneous respiration has been abolished by use of a muscle relaxant, is to hyperventilate the patient using a minute volume considerably in excess of the patient's calculated requirements.

3. The third and perhaps least satisfactory method of determining that respiration is adequate is to exclude signs of hypoxia and of carbon dioxide retention.

HYPOXIA is normally recognised by the appearance of cyanosis. It must, however, be remembered that before cyanosis is visible 5 G. per cent. of reduced haemoglobin must be present. This means that, even allowing that the patient has a high level of haemoglobin, about 15 G. per cent., the oxygen saturation will have fallen to about 66 per cent. before cyanosis is detected. The other signs normally associated with hypoxia are a rise in heart rate, a slight rise in blood pressure and, where the patient is breathing, tachypnoea.

SIGNS OF CARBON DIOXIDE RETENTION normally appear when the arterial carbon dioxide tension has reached levels about double the normal, that is between 80 and 100 mm. Hg. They are as follows:—

(*a*) The skin becomes hot, flushed and moist, the so-called " boiled lobster syndrome ", because of the similarity in colour to that of a freshly boiled lobster. These signs are caused by dilatation of the arterioles and capillaries by a local action of the carbon dioxide.

(*b*) Central action of the carbon dioxide on the vasomotor centre results in vasoconstriction of the larger vessels, in particular the splanchnic vessels, which causes a rise in blood pressure.

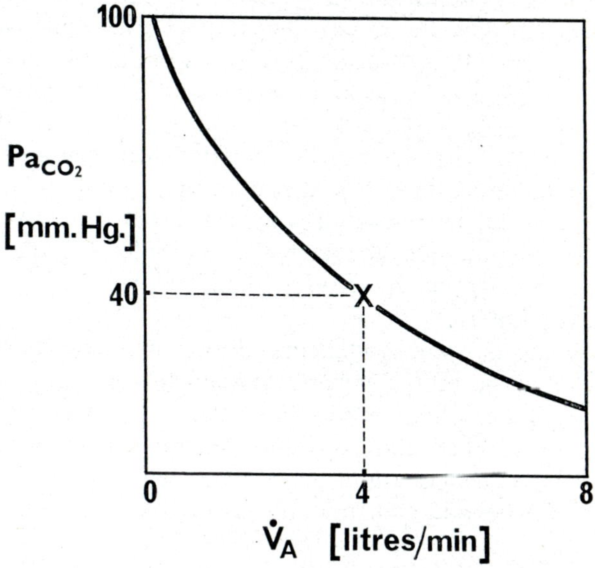

FIG. 73

This graph illustrates the relationship between alveolar ventilation ($\dot{V}_A$) and arterial carbon dioxide tension ($P_{a\ CO_2}$).

A resting alveolar ventilatory level of 4 litres/minute, in the normal patient, ensures an arterial carbon dioxide tension of around 40 mm. Hg.

(*c*) The heart rate rises in the early stages of carbon dioxide retention and only in the later stages, when the conducting mechanism is poisoned, does the rate slow before the heart fails.

(*d*) The respiratory response to carbon dioxide is an increase in depth and/or rate of respiration, but the anaesthetist must not depend too much on these signs, since it is often in circumstances where the patient cannot respond by increase in rate or depth of respiration that carbon dioxide retention takes place. Frequently, respiration will have been depressed by central or peripheral mechanisms and it is when this compensation breaks down that trouble is to be expected.

(*e*) It is often noted during emergence from anaesthesia, when carbon dioxide tension is allowed to increase, that bleeding from skin edges increases and during anaesthesia this may be taken as an indication that carbon dioxide is inadvertently increasing. It must be stressed that this is only significant when bleeding takes place from small vessels and that bleeding from major vessels is a surgical problem and not an anaesthetic sign.

(*f*) A sign of carbon dioxide retention, which is of importance to the anaesthetist post-operatively, is that confusion, restlessness and the onset of unconsciousness may be found when carbon dioxide is retained in considerable quantities. Often, in retrospect, this is a good indication of the onset of respiratory failure.

While it is now recognised that during spontaneous respiration with many of the volatile anaesthetics, oxygen tensions below ideal levels and carbon dioxide tensions of almost twice normal are reached and apparently tolerated by healthy individuals, early recognition of inadequate respiration is desirable and should be an indication for assisted or controlled ventilation.

The importance of recognising inadequate respiration goes far beyond the practice of anaesthesia. Any doctor no matter where he or she practises will encounter patients whose respiration is, temporarily at least, inadequate. These may be patients suffering from an overdose of barbiturates or other drugs, patients who have had a cerebro-vascular accident or head injury, and patients suffering from post-operative respiratory depression. In addition, patients with chronic obstructive lung disease may, during an episode of acute infection, develop respiratory insufficiency.

The signs of inadequate respiration, as described in this chapter, may be found in some of these patients to co-exist with signs suggestive of respiratory obstruction. It is sometimes not appreciated that it is the respiratory obstruction, the inadequate respiration and pulmonary complications which are the cause of death in many of these patients. Recognition of the condition and treatment either on the spot, or, in an appropriate unit in the case of long term treatment, is often life saving.

CIRCULATORY COMPLICATIONS

Complications affecting the circulation during anaesthesia may be considered in two main groups. These are (1) complications detected by changes in blood pressure and (2) complications detected by changes in heart rate and rhythm.

Changes in Blood Pressure

The blood pressure may rise, fall or fluctuate widely.

HYPOTENSION can be due to a wide variety of causes during anaesthesia. Some of these are associated with central depression of the vasomotor centre, resulting in vasodilatation; some with depression of the myocardium resulting in decreased cardiac output; some with diminished venous return to the heart and others with blood loss.

It is not unusual for a patient, having had premedication, to come to the anaesthetic room with a systolic blood pressure up to 25 mm. Hg. below the resting level, as measured in the ward. This is not an unexpected phenomenon in that the blood pressure may also fall as much as 25 mm. Hg during normal sleep and the patient who is resting quietly after premedication may obviously be expected to show similar changes. Occasionally, the fall in blood pressure is more marked, particularly with some premedications such as phenothiazine drugs and pethidine. After the administration of thiopentone and during the maintenance of anaesthesia, particularly before surgical stimuli have been applied, it is again not unusual to find the blood pressure depressed below the resting level. After surgery has commenced, however, it is common to find the blood pressure restored to a level not far removed from the patient's resting value, although in some cases it may settle at a level lower than normal.

Hypotension during anaesthesia carries the risk of cerebral and myocardial damage from hypoxia or arterial thrombosis. The oxygenation of these and other tissues does not depend entirely on the level of blood pressure. Vasodilatation, arterial oxygen content, the blood flow—which may vary from organ to organ—and pooling of blood in dependent parts are all important factors. A further complication, where low blood pressures are maintained for a long period, is that the renal and hepatic circulation may be inadequate with consequent damage to these organs.

The critical level of systolic blood pressure at which such damage may occur is a matter of some doubt, although it is widely recognised that renal damage may ensue when the blood pressure is allowed to fall below 60 mm. Hg systolic. Many patients, in fact, undergo anaesthesia with systolic blood pressures ranging between 80 and 100 mm. Hg without apparent ill effect post-operatively, and, indeed, if the blood pressure is observed in all cases, it is surprising how often the pressure runs along at such levels, although no measures have been taken to lower it at all. Where possible, however, it is desirable to maintain the systolic blood pressure reasonably close to the normal resting pressure.

THE TREATMENT OF HYPOTENSION will naturally depend on its cause.

1. Where it is thought to be due to depression by drugs such as thiopentone, halothane or other potent anaesthetic agents, the concentration of these agents should be reduced if possible. In addition, whenever possible, a high concentration of oxygen should be administered and, in the case of halothane, if there is an associated bradycardia, intravenous atropine, 0·6 mg., may raise the pressure. The administration of vasopressors such as methoxamine 5-15 mg. intramuscularly, may be necessary.

2. When ventilation is controlled, by manual or mechanical inflation of the lungs, the changes in intrathoracic pressure abolish the respiratory pump action which allows the heart and great veins to fill during inspiration. This potentially harmful effect of intermittent positive pressure ventilation is discussed more fully in Chapter XI. In general, it is wise to inflate the lungs at the lowest possible pressure consistent with adequate ventilation.

Sometimes the blood pressure will fall during positive pressure ventilation, when the muscle relaxant is wearing off, and greater pressure than before is required to inflate the lungs.

This can be corrected by a further dose of muscle relaxant. While some fall in blood pressure may accompany the administration of *d*-tubocurarine, usually this is only of serious degree when large doses of the drug are administered.

3. Hypotension due to blood loss is treated by blood transfusion or, as a temporary measure, by infusion of plasma, Macrodex or Rheomacrodex.

THE USE OF VASOCONSTRICTORS is limited. Where blood has been lost, the peripheral circulation is normally constricted as a physiological response to haemorrhage. Clearly further vasoconstriction is either impossible or certainly undesirable, in that it may well result in extremely poor tissue perfusion, which, when the circulation returns to normal, results in severe metabolic acidosis.

HYPERTENSION is a complication sometimes found during anaesthesia and it is normally indicative of one of two conditions. In the first place, underventilation may be taking place and the patient retaining carbon dioxide and becoming hypoxic. This diagnosis may be confirmed by measuring the depth of respiration. If this is inadequate, assisted or controlled ventilation should be instituted or increased. Another cause of hypertension during anaesthesia is inadequate analgesia with the patient reacting to surgical stimuli. This can be confirmed by looking for the other signs of reflex activity, and treated by administering supplementary analgesia, either by adding volatile agents to the mixture or by intravenous administration of small doses, 10-25 mg., of pethidine.

A rare cause of severe hypertension during anaesthesia is a phaeochromocytoma.

Hypotension or hypertension are more marked as a rule where the resting blood pressure is raised. These hypertensive subjects are also more susceptible to the cardiovascular effects of drugs, mechanical ventilation and to blood loss. They are very sensitive to vasopressor drugs and also show marked rises in blood pressure when analgesia is inadequate. The anaesthetic for a hypertensive patient must therefore be conducted in such a manner as to avoid wide fluctuations in blood pressure which may be tolerable in patients without cardiovascular disease.

Changes in Heart Rate and Rhythm

TACHYCARDIA may follow the administration of some drugs used in anaesthesia. It may be a physiological response to hypotension or may be caused by drugs with vagolytic effects such as atropine, pethidine or gallamine (Flaxedil). The administration of ether is often accompanied by tachycardia.

As a result, heart rates of about 100/minute are not uncommon during otherwise apparently uneventful anaesthesia but care must, however, be taken to exclude the possibility that tachycardia is due to haemorrhage and it has been mentioned previously as a sign both of inadequate analgesia and of inadequate respiration.

Where it is found as an accompaniment of certain of the drugs mentioned, it has perhaps to be accepted, but when it results from haemorrhage, inadequate ventilation or inadequate analgesia, confirmatory signs should be sought and the appropriate treatment instituted.

BRADYCARDIA is found after certain drugs have been administered. It may follow a dose of hyoscine (Scopolamine) and is found when cyclopropane or halothane are used as the main agents. It is probably advisable to give atropine before these inhalational agents and, if bradycardia is severe during anaesthesia, the intravenous administration of atropine, 0·6 mg., is recommended. Bradycardia may also accompany the use of intravenous suxamethonium and certainly after a second and subsequent doses it may be profound, even to the extent of no heart beat being palpable for up to seven seconds. Again this can be minimised by prophylactic administration of atropine and by restricting the second and further doses of suxamethonium to a maximum of 25 mg.

CARDIAC ARRHYTHMIAS of various types occur during anaesthesia and are particularly associated with the administration of halogenated anaesthetics such as chloroform, trichloroethylene and halothane and also with cyclopropane. Many reasons have been advanced for their occurrence but it is now generally agreed that they occur principally when the arterial carbon dioxide tension is high during the administration of these agents. Although it has been shown that arrhythmias are frequently present, without any great harm resulting, they should always be considered potentially dangerous and adequate ventilation must be maintained. If this does not cause the arrhythmias to disappear, the concentration of the anaesthetic agent should be reduced or a change be made to another agent.

The arrhythmias may, of themselves, be a sign of severe carbon dioxide retention and oxygen lack. Again ventilation should be assisted until it is adequate.

Where the heart beat is absent and a pulse cannot be felt in a major vessel such as the carotid, a provisional diagnosis of a *cardiac arrest* should be made and confirmatory signs sought (p. 148). It must be stressed that such a diagnosis is made only when pulsation in a major vessel cannot be felt and not when pulsation cannot be obtained in the radial or facial arteries. During anaesthesia, for a variety of reasons, such as posture, the position of a head harness or indeed vasoconstriction, pulsation in these smaller arteries may be difficult to feel. When no carotid pulse is felt, the apex beat should be rapidly checked, by a stethoscope or by palpation, to see if any sounds or pulsation can be heard or felt there. If the abdomen is open, the surgeon should be asked to palpate the aorta. In the absence of pulsation in a major vessel and the absence of heart beat or pulsation in the aorta, a cardiac arrest should be presumed.

At this point, a carefully organised plan must be put into effect, as, within three or four minutes of cessation of circulation, irreparable damage to the brain will take place. Where cardiac massage is instituted, the anaesthetist should ensure that ventilation of the lungs with 100 per cent. oxygen is continued throughout the attempts at resuscitation. The problem of cardiac arrest and the methods of dealing with it, both by external cardiac compression and direct cardiac massage, are considered in greater detail in the section dealing with resuscitation (p. 197).

So important is it to recognise instantly the occurrence of cardiac arrest that many authorities consider that monitoring of the pulse by instruments, attached usually to the finger tip and recording visually or audibly each heart beat, is highly desirable during anaesthesia. Such an instrument is shown in Figure 74. This does not of course take the place of an electrocardiograph but it is not at present practicable to have an electrocardiograph attached to every patient in the theatre.

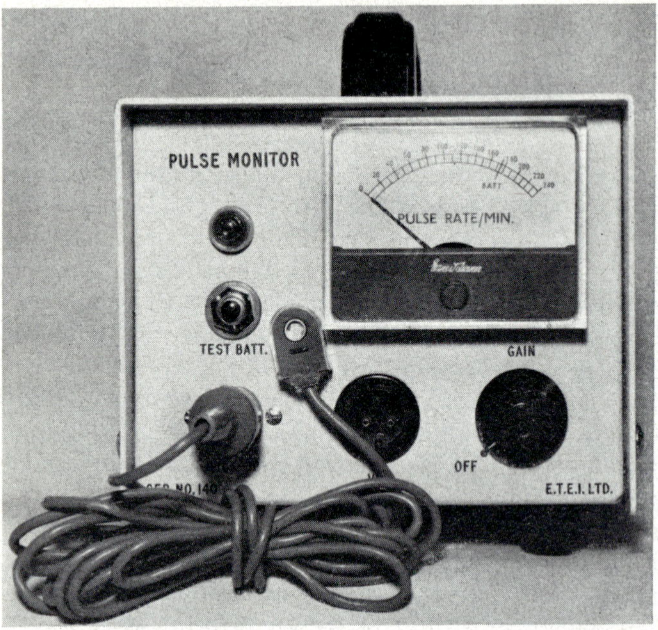

FIG. 74
The M.I.E. pulse monitor. The photoelectric sensor is attached to the end of the cable.

Some pulse monitoring devices have, however, the disadvantage that during surgery they tend to pick up extraneous movements of the limb to which they are attached and during operations when vasoconstriction takes place the record of each beat may be extremely faint. Unfortunately it is under such circumstances that their importance is greatest. Whichever method is used, whether electrocardiograph, pulse monitor or careful palpation of the pulse at regular intervals, the anaesthetist should always be alert to any alteration in heart rate or rhythm.

VOMITING AND REGURGITATION

Vomiting and regurgitation may take place during maintenance of anaesthesia as during induction. Again the best treatment is prevention. In addition, it is customary to insert a cuffed endotracheal tube as soon as practicable after induction and so ensure that, if vomiting or regurgitation takes place, stomach contents will not be inhaled into the lungs.

There are, however, occasions where there is no apparent indication that vomiting or regurgitation is to be expected during anaesthesia and where precautions have not been taken to deal with this hazard.

VOMITING can be recognised by the actual movement of the patient in active vomiting and is often preceded by lightening of the anaesthetic and a period of shallow, possibly irregular, breathing.

REGURGITATION is of course a silent process where fluid wells up from the stomach with no outward signs that it is imminent. Sometimes the first indication of disaster is the rattling of fluid in the airway as the patient breathes; or the first indication, during lighter anaesthesia, may be a laryngeal spasm. Transparent anaesthetic masks have been designed so that vomitus can be seen at once. In addition, in patients liable to vomit, e.g. obstetric cases and casualties, the mask should never be strapped to the face so that, if vomiting does take place, treatment can be rapidly instituted.

THE TREATMENT is in the first place to lower the patient's head or turn it to one side. Thereafter the vomitus should be aspirated or swabbed from the pharynx. During light anaesthesia this may be all that is required and, if the anaesthetic is continued with the head down and to the side, regurgitated material is unlikely to pass into the trachea. If inhalation of vomitus has taken place then steps should be taken to aspirate the trachea immediately, either through an endotracheal tube or by bronchoscopy. The use of a head down posture may assist these measures.

When only a small quantity of gastric content has been aspirated Mendelson's syndrome may develop, characterised by acute bronchospasm and by circulatory collapse. Being liquid it passes into the distal parts of the lungs and aspiration through a bronchoscope or through an endotracheal tube is not usually successful, and, as the patient is already in a grave state because of acute bronchospasm and consequent hypoxia, tracheobronchial suction, by causing further hypoxia, may be frankly dangerous and even lethal. Oxygen 100 per cent.

should be given by intermittent positive pressure ventilation, if necessary; anti-spasmodic agents such as aminophylline may be administered and large doses of hydrocortisone should be given intravenously in the treatment of this condition. Bronchial lavage perhaps of segments of the lung with sterile buffered saline may be of value. In addition, support of the circulation by vasoconstrictors or the administration of plasma is important. This complication carries a high mortality rate.

The late treatment of these complications is dealt with in Chapter X.

MALIGNANT HYPERPYREXIA. Recently, reports have appeared of patients developing high fever and increasing muscle tone during anaesthesia. The aetiology is uncertain and the mortality rate high. Treatment is directed towards relief of the severe metabolic acidosis and hyperkalaemia which occur.

CHAPTER X

RECOVERY ROOM—AFTER CARE OF PATIENTS

All patients should be observed during the post-operative period, ideally in a centralised recovery room beside the operating theatre. The length of stay in this room will depend on the condition of the patient and the nature of the surgical procedure and anaesthesia. Close observation and care of patients during the crucial post-operative period when consciousness and reflexes may still be impaired results in economy of nursing and medical personnel and apparatus. Where such facilities are not available some compromise is necessary but it should be possible to nurse major surgical, seriously ill and emergency cases through the recovery period in a side ward near the theatre or in a screened-off section of the general ward. Whatever the local arrangement, it is essential that all nurses and medical staff engaged in post-operative care should be trained specially for this work and be capable of carrying out certain emergency resuscitative measures.

COMPLICATIONS OF ANAESTHESIA

The complications requiring the special attention of the recovery room staff readily fall into three groups:—

1. *Respiratory*: Obstruction of the airway; respiratory inadequacy and respiratory arrest.
2. *Circulatory*: Hypotension; cardiac irregularities and cardiac arrest.
3. *Gastro-intestinal*: Vomiting and regurgitation of stomach contents.

These main groups may frequently overlap, e.g. a patient while still recovering from anaesthesia may regurgitate, inhale gastric contents and suffer respiratory obstruction. Untreated, this could lead to cardiac arrest and death.

We will now consider these complications in more detail, describing their mechanism, their recognition and appropriate treatment.

1. Respiratory Complications

Obstruction of the Airway. The commonest respiratory complication, in the immediate post-operative period, is obstruction of the patient's upper airway. The three commonest causes are (1) the tongue falling back against the posterior wall of the pharynx when the patient is supine, (2) the presence of foreign material in the pharynx, and (3) laryngeal spasm. Respiratory obstruction can again be diagnosed when movements of the chest and abdomen are exaggerated but very little air passes through the nose or mouth with the patient becoming increasingly cyanosed. Laryngeal spasm often produces a " crowing " noise as air passes through the constricted larynx. It is worth remembering that *noisy breathing is always obstructed breathing, but not all obstructed breathing is noisy.*

Treatment. 1. Secure a clear airway immediately. This is usually accomplished by pulling the lower jaw upwards and forwards thus pulling the tongue away from the posterior pharyngeal wall. Only rarely should it be necessary to grip the tongue and pull it forward with forceps. Suction may be required to remove any obstruction, e.g. mucus. Oxygen may have to be administered but is quite useless unless the airway is already clear.

2. If no improvement follows these manoeuvres quickly GET HELP.

Respiratory Insufficiency. Despite an unobstructed upper airway, some patients may not breathe deeply enough to ensure adequate respiratory exchange in the alveoli. Any interference with this mechanism results in hypoxia and carbon dioxide accumulation (Figs. 73 and 75). This may occur for many reasons, viz.

(*a*) A common cause is obstruction of the smaller airways or bronchi.

(*b*) Depression of the respiratory centre following head injuries or cerebrovascular accidents, or the prolonged effects of anaesthetic agents.

(*c*) Disease of or damage to the nervous pathways to the muscles of respiration, e.g. poliomyelitis.

(*d*) Weakness of the muscles of respiration as in myasthenia gravis, or when the action of relaxant drugs has not been fully reversed at the end of the operation.

(*e*) Removal of lung tissue, as in lobectomy or pneumonectomy.

(*f*) Pre-existing lung disease, e.g. chronic bronchitis or emphysema.

(*g*) Constriction of the chest wall or abdomen interfering with normal expansion during breathing. This may be the result of pre-existing disease of the thoracic cage, e.g. ankylosing

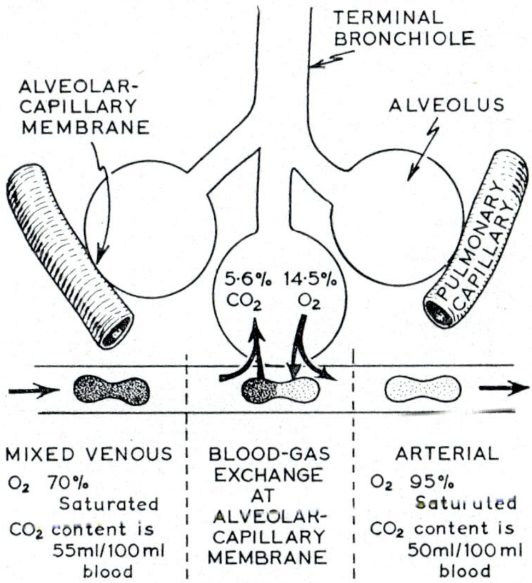

FIG. 75

The alveolar-capillary diagram: this diagram demonstrates the blood-gas changes which take place during normal respiration as the blood passes through the lungs.

spondylitis, or a simpler cause sometimes found is the application of too tight a dressing following operation. The recognition of inadequate respiration has already been discussed (p. 131).

In addition if the patient has previously been conscious, respiratory inadequacy may be evidenced by increasing restlessness, confusion, drowsiness and eventual coma.

Treatment. Having secured a clear airway, the next step, no matter what the underlying cause of the respiratory inadequacy, must always be to assist the patient's own inadequate efforts. Increasing the amount of oxygen in the inspired air alone rarely results in improvement. Many simple devices are now available to augment the patient's respiration. These enable the doctor or nurse to administer atmospheric air or oxygen by intermittent compression of a bag or bellows, e.g. Ambu resuscitator, Lucas bellows, etc. (Fig. 76).

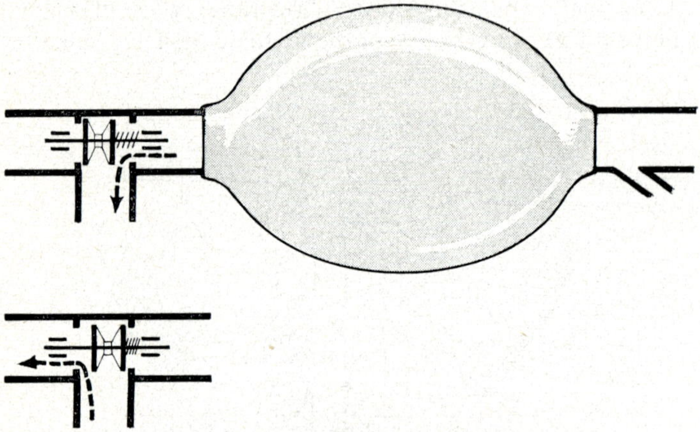

FIG. 76

The Ambu resuscitator: additional oxygen may be fed into the bag through the small side tube at the right of the picture thus enriching the air which is driven into the patient's lungs when the bag is compressed. On the left of the illustration is the non-return valve connected to a mask or endotracheal tube by the vertical limb. The patient's expirations are delivered to the atmosphere through the horizontal limb of the valve.

No recovery room should be without one or other of these simple devices and all staff should be skilled in their use. When no apparatus is immediately available the physician must resort to other measures to support the patient's failing or absent respiration. The simplest and most effective of these is the technique of expired air resuscitation or mouth-to-mouth breathing. A detailed description of this method is given in Chapter XII.

2. Circulatory Complications

When considering *circulatory changes* following anaesthesia, it is important to remember the significance of alterations in the patient's colour. Pallor or flushing in the absence of other signs of shock or of inadequate respiration, may be quite normal. Cyanosis *always* calls for urgent treatment.

The temperature of patients returning to a recovery room post-operatively may often be found to be slightly sub-normal. While it is important to prevent such patients shivering, only exceptionally should heat be applied, as this results in diversion of the blood from the vital organs to the skin.

PULSE. The pulse rate should be carefully observed during the immediate post-operative period.

A moderate tachycardia (80-100/min.) commonly follows major surgery but a persistent tachycardia, particularly if it is increasing, should always be regarded as a danger sign, indicating perhaps haemorrhage or inadequate respiration.

BLOOD PRESSURE. Following a major operation the blood pressure may be below the pre-operative value, as a result of the surgery itself and of the continuing action of drugs administered by the anaesthetist. A systolic blood pressure of about 20 mm. Hg below the pre-operative value can often be accepted, but where it continues to fall or to rise unduly an explanation should be sought. All patients who have had a general anaesthetic, and some to whom a regional analgesic has been given, are liable to hypotension and even sudden cardiac arrest if they are roughly handled or put in the sitting-up position (postural hypotension); they should be moved gently from trolley to bed and kept flat (or in the tonsillar position) until recovery is complete. In special cases, the bed may be tilted to a moderate head-down position for the first hour or two.

Frequent blood pressure readings are time consuming and not usually necessary (e.g. not more often than every 20-30 minutes). Close observation of colour change in the skin, level of consciousness and pulse rate provide the necessary information in most patients.

VENOUS PRESSURE. The measurement of central venous pressure is frequently made by the anaesthetist in theatre, particularly in cases of severe injuries or during surgery involving a large loss of blood. The central venous pressure is a sensitive index of changes in circulating blood volume and begins to fall before changes in pulse rate or systemic arterial pressure can be detected. Measurements may continue to be made during the recovery period as a guide to further blood or plasma requirements.

Cardiac irregularities in the post-operative period should always be reported to the anaesthetist. Atrial fibrillation in elderly patients may occur following major surgery and its onset is often accompanied by a fall in blood pressure. Bursts of extrasystoles (dropped-beats) may herald the onset of ventricular fibrillation and cardiac arrest. The precise diagnosis of cardiac irregularities usually depends on the ECG and therefore the earlier their occurrence is reported the better.

CARDIAC ARREST. The most sudden and dramatic of all emergencies with which the recovery room personnel may have to deal is that of " cardiac arrest ". This may follow untreated respiratory inadequacy or a period of persistent hypotension due to any cause, but it can frequently occur without warning. Any patients who are especially " at risk " e.g. those with some degree of heart-block pre-operatively, should be indicated to the staff by the anaesthetist. In healthy adults, the sensitive tissue of the brain will only survive the results of circulatory standstill and acute hypoxia for a period of about three minutes. The immediate recognition of this condition is therefore of the utmost importance if resuscitation is to be successful.

Signs of "Apparent Cardiac Arrest". The term " apparent cardiac arrest " is used deliberately since, if the cardiac action and circulation are so poor that the following signs are present, then immediate treatment is required even if the heart has not quite stopped.

The signs are three in number:—

Pallor or cyanosis of the skin, i.e. a sudden deterioration of the skin colour.

Absence of palpable carotid pulses in the neck. N.B. not the radial pulses as these are often difficult to feel.

Rapidly dilating pupils. This is a most reliable sign of cerebral hypoxia.

Two secondary signs should be noted.

Loss of consciousness. This, of course, only if the patient was not already unconscious.

Cessation of respiration. If action is not taken quickly enough following cardiac arrest then respiratory arrest will follow.

Treatment of Cardiac Arrest. If these signs are present, *immediate action* is required. Until recently this would have taken the form of direct cardiac massage but, since 1960, a new method of indirect or external cardiac compression is to be preferred, in the first instance. This method may only fill the gap in time until "direct massage" can be instituted or may actually itself be sufficient to restore cardiac action and circulation completely. The technique of external cardiac compression is described in Chapter XII.

3. Gastro-intestinal Complications

It is necessary to distinguish between vomiting which is an active process and regurgitation which is a passive and more insidious complication. Regurgitation is seldom accompanied by any outward signs or sounds and occurs when the patient is at a deeper level of unconsciousness and his cough reflex is absent or less active than normal. Unless adequate precautions have been taken inhalation of the gastric contents will certainly occur. The vomiting patient on the other hand can usually cough vigorously and the vomitus unless excessive in quantity can be expelled without danger of inhalation.

This complication is most likely to occur if the stomach has not been emptied adequately before operation, if there was vomiting pre-operatively, or if the nature of the illness results in delayed gastric emptying.

Certain anaesthetic agents predispose to nausea and vomiting in the post-operative period, e.g. cyclopropane and ether, but with modern anaesthetic techniques vomiting from this latter cause is uncommon.

Inhalation of gastric contents can result in sudden death from drowning or in acute hypoxia from laryngeal or bronchial spasm. A late result may be the development of pulmonary collapse, pneumonia or lung abscess. One group of patients, in whom inhalation of foreign material is particularly likely, deserves special mention. When the pharynx and vocal cords have been anaesthetised by topical application of an analgesic agent, e.g. lignocaine 4 per cent., to facilitate endoscopy, the loss of sensation often exceeds the actual operating time by up to two hours. Thus fluids or solids must not be given until the analgesic has ceased to act, lest they are inhaled when the patient attempts to swallow. A simple label on the patient's forehead, indicating that a topical analgesic has been used, is a useful precaution.

Treatment. The best treatment of the condition is prevention. Wherever possible, the stomach should be emptied preoperatively. Even when a gastric tube is left in place after operation, regurgitation may still take place alongside the tube, particularly if drainage is not free, e.g. if a clamp or spigot is left on the upper end of the tube.

The dangers of vomiting and regurgitation may be prevented to a large extent by correct posturing of the patient in bed, i.e. " the tonsillar position " (Fig. 52).

If vomiting or regurgitation does occur:—

1. Keep the head low. This ensures that all the material will flow out of the mouth and not enter the respiratory tract.

2. Clear the mouth and pharynx with swabs or suction.

3. Having cleared the airway, ensure that respiration is adequate. If cyanosis persists, administer oxygen.

4. If there is evidence that stomach contents have actually been inhaled then pulmonary lavage may be indicated. Acute pulmonary oedema may follow inhalation of even a small quantity of acid material and should be treated with oxygen, assistance to ventilation, steroid therapy and antibiotics.

4. Renal Complications

It has been said that one unnecessary risk to the critically ill patient could be avoided if as much attention was paid to measurement of urine flow as to changes in pulse rate. Normally functioning kidneys are essential not only to body water and electrolyte balance but also to acid base homeostasis. Incipient renal failure may pass unnoticed in the immediate post-operative period unless there is a proper understanding of its mechanisms and a recognition of the ' high risk ' situations in which it is likely to occur.

A simple classification of renal failure is:

(*a*) Pre-renal.

(*b*) Intrinsic.

(*c*) Post-renal.

We are concerned here only with the pre-renal and intrinsic types. In the pre-renal type of failure which is commonly met with in the surgical patient, treatment consists of adequate restoration of the circulating blood volume, replacement of fluids and correction of electrolyte deficiencies. This will usually result in a return of normal urine flow from the previous oliguric state. Uncorrected or undetected, the pre-renal type of failure can progress to the intrinsic variety which has in times past been referred to as acute tubular necrosis. Failure to secure a normal urine flow following restoration of the circulating blood volume normally indicates that intrinsic failure is already established. Even at this stage the situation may be reversible if a diuretic such as 20 per cent. Mannitol is given intravenously. Failure to respond to this therapy is an indication for further treatment by the renal physicians which may be conservative or may consist of repeated peritoneal dialysis or haemodialysis until normal renal function returns.

To summarise, the predisposing factors are:—

(*a*) Reduced renal blood flow due to a reduction in circulating blood, plasma or water and electrolytes.

(*b*) Metabolic acidosis which, for example, is almost invariably present in the shocked patient.

(*c*) Excessive circulating haemoglobin or myoglobin as commonly found in grave multiple injuries.

(*d*) Sepsis.

(*e*) Surgery on the aorta at or above the level of the renal vessels.

Close observation of these patients in the immediate post-operative phase is essential and should consist of hourly urine volume measurement along with blood pressure and central venous pressure measurements. Frequent blood gas analysis to detect any metabolic acidosis is important as are the measurement of urine and plasma osmolalities.

The initial treatment is outlined below but the early recognition of the condition and collaboration with the renal physicians is of the first importance.

Treatment. (*a*) Maintenance of normal blood volume.

(*b*) Correction of fluid and electrolyte deficiencies.

(*c*) Intravenous 20 per cent. Mannitol (two or three doses maximum).

CARE OF SPECIAL CASES IN THE RECOVERY ROOM

There are additional points to observe in the management of patients who have undergone certain special types of surgery or anaesthesia.

1. Epidural and Subarachnoid Analgesia

These analgesic techniques interfere with three important functions of the patient's normal defence mechanism and this state of affairs often persists well into the recovery period.

ANALGESIA. The regions of the body, and particularly the skin, served by the nerves which have been blocked as they leave the subarachnoid (spinal) or epidural spaces, may still be partially or completely affected post-operatively. So far as the skin is concerned the patient will not respond normally to pain, heat or cold. Contact with a rough projection on the bed or a hot-water bottle will therefore result in injury (traumatic ulceration or burns).

REFLEXES. The normal postural reflexes will be depressed. These reflexes normally prevent over-stretching of muscles or over-extension of joints. Damage can result if the limbs are allowed to remain in abnormal positions for long periods.

The use of " ripple mattresses " is of great assistance in the prevention of bed sores in any patient where the one posture is, of necessity, maintained for a long time (Fig. 77).

SYMPATHETIC BLOCKADE. Under sympathetic blockade the normal control of the peripheral blood vessels which helps to maintain the blood pressure at the normal levels is temporarily lost. Thus, blood pools in the dependent parts of the body and a severe fall in blood pressure occurs. Therefore, patients under the influence of a " spinal " or epidural analgesic must be nursed in the recumbent position and occasionally in the head-down position until the normal tone returns to the cardiovascular system.

There are other points to observe in the management of such cases:—

(*a*) *Headache*. Not infrequently this follows subarachnoid analgesia and its causation is obscure. However, it is well known that headache is much commoner in patients who have not been nursed in the supine position for at least 12 hours after the operation.

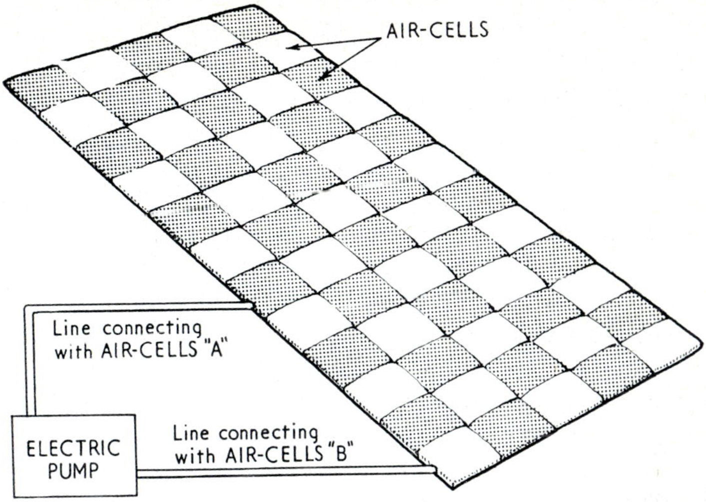

FIG. 77

The "ripple" mattress: One design of the mattress is shown diagrammatically. The electric pump automatically inflates air-cells A and air-cells B alternately thus avoiding constant pressure at any one point on the patient's back.

(*b*) *Acute Retention of Urine*. This can occur particularly in older men with prostatic enlargement. However, while the analgesic effect persists, the distended bladder does not cause undue discomfort. The abdomen therefore should be examined regularly for any sign of bladder distension, and catheterisation may be required.

(*c*) *Sterility*. Particular care must be taken of patients in whom a continuous epidural analgesia is being maintained post-operatively. The staff may be instructed to make the intermittent injections at certain intervals and *absolute* sterility is essential. A new technique, using a paediatric intravenous set with burette, avoids this danger to some extent.

2. Induced Hypotensive Anaesthesia

Some surgical procedures are facilitated if bleeding in the field of operation is reduced to a minimum by lowering the blood pressure deliberately during anaesthesia, e.g. brain surgery, micro-surgery of the middle ear and plastic surgery.

Hypotension may be induced in one of two ways:—

(*a*) By epidural or subarachnoid analgesia.

(*b*) By the intravenous injection of ganglion blocking drugs such as trimetaphan (Arfonad).

The loss of vasomotor tone (i.e. dilatation of the blood vessels) produced by these methods may last well into the recovery phase and although the patient may have become fully conscious, he is still very likely to suffer a severe fall in blood pressure if allowed to sit up. Frequent pulse and blood pressure recording is therefore of the greatest importance in these patients, until the hypotensive effect wears off.

3. Induced Hypothermia

This technique is usually confined to cardiovascular and neurosurgical procedures, or following severe head injuries. The patient's body temperature is lowered to between 29°C. and 32°C. (normal body temperature 37°C.) and active rewarming of such cases is carried out in the recovery room until the body temperature is about 36°C. Rewarming is carried out with electric blankets, special mattresses which contain circulating warm water, or by a fan blowing warm air over the body surface. Although the process is always closely supervised by the anaesthetist, the recovery room staff has an important part to play. The recording of temperature at frequent intervals, in addition to pulse, blood pressure and respiratory rate, is usually the responsibility of the nurse. A few words of explanation about temperature recording in these cases may be useful at this point.

" Body " temperature is a meaningless phrase unless the site at which the recording is made is indicated, e.g. rectum, oesophagus, nasopharynx or axilla. Commonly during rewarming the rectal or oesophageal temperature is monitored by specially designed continuously recording thermometers (Figs. 78 and 79). The mercury clinical thermometer is not suitable. The temperature is read at frequent intervals, e.g. five minutes until a return to normal is achieved. Figure 80 shows the changes in oesophageal temperature in a patient, during the whole pre-operative cooling procedure and the post-operative warming phase.

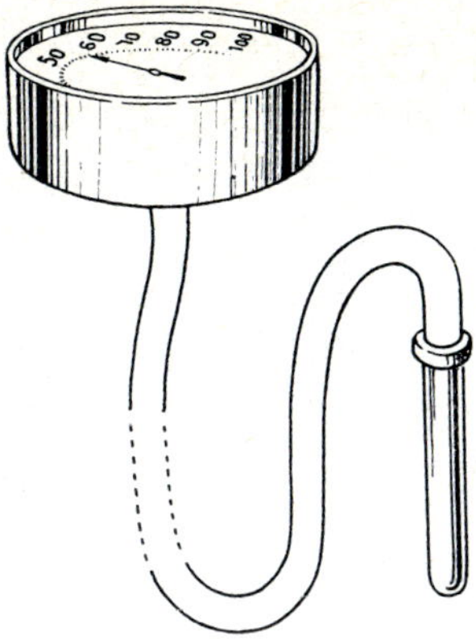

FIG. 78

A rectal thermometer. The sensing device is a reservoir bulb filled with mercury. This is connected to the gauge by a flexible capillary tube. The probe is left *in situ* and frequent readings can be made.

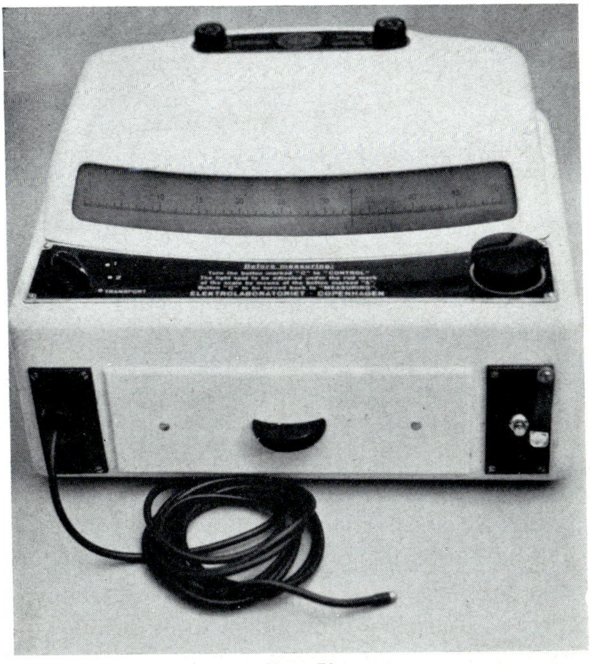

FIG. 79

A recording thermometer with an oesophageal lead attached.

Special attention must be paid to the skin during rewarming to avoid contact burns and pressure sores.

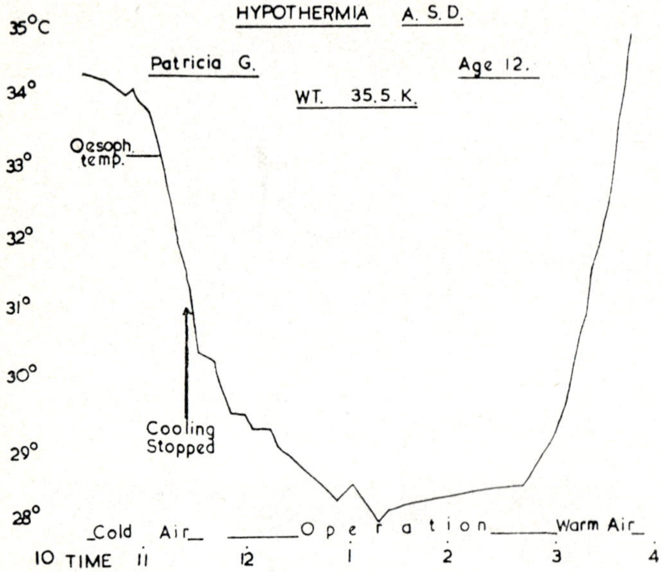

FIG. 80

This temperature chart shows the oesophageal temperature changes during the repair of an atrial septal defect (A.S.D.) in a child weighing 35·5 kilograms.

4. Endoscopies

The diagnostic procedures of laryngoscopy, bronchoscopy and oesophagoscopy are frequently carried out under topical analgesia, with or without a general anaesthetic as well. Lignocaine in a 4 per cent. solution is commonly employed and its analgesic action may last up to two hours. During this period there is a loss of sensation in the mouth, oropharynx and larynx and the cough reflex is depressed. It is obvious that two dangers must be avoided in the recovery room:—

(*a*) Any solids or liquids given orally may enter the lungs.

(*b*) Hot liquids may cause burns to the anaesthetised area.

For a period of at least three hours from the start of anaesthesia, no fluids or solids are given to these patients despite the fact that they may be fully conscious and co-operative.

Due to the absence of the cough reflex, secretions tend to accumulate in the mouth and airway and patients must be encouraged to cough them up or, if necessary, they must be removed by gentle suction. The use of the tonsillar position in bed, even when the patient is fully conscious, has much to recommend it.

5. Restless Patients

Restlessness, during recovery from anaesthesia, is common and the diagnosis and treatment of the underlying cause is worthy of mention. Too often such restlessness is interpreted only as a need for a sedative or analgesic. It is essential that the cause be accurately identified and sedation must be withheld until this has been done. The following are some of the possible causes of post-operative restlessness:—

(*a*) *Inadequate Respiration*: This can be diagnosed with certainty if signs of hypoxia or carbon dioxide retention are present (p. 132).

(*b*) *Haemorrhage*: A fall in blood pressure with tachycardia is strongly suggestive of hidden bleeding.

(*c*) *Pain other than Wound Pain*: This may result from a full bladder, pins in the dressings puncturing the skin, contact with hot-water bottles etc.

When other causes have been excluded, and only then, is it safe to assume that pain at the site of the operation is responsible and an analgesic is indicated, e.g. morphine 10-15 mg. Occasionally, in the absence of pain, a simple sedative to allay nervousness is sufficient, e.g. a barbiturate such as amylobarbitone (Amytal) or quinalbarbitone (Seconal) 100-200 mg.

6. Post-Thoracotomy Patients

Certain post-operative complications may occur in patients who have undergone thoracotomy. The two most dangerous are unrecognised bleeding inside the chest resulting in a *haemothorax,* and air inside the chest escaping from a damaged area of lung resulting in *pneumothorax*. The presence of blood or air in quantity within the pleural cavity causes collapse of the underlying lung resulting in inadequate ventilation. To prevent these dangers a drain is usually inserted into the pleural cavity at the end of the operation. The drain is a special type and its open end passes into a bottle and is kept under the surface of some suitable sterile liquid (Fig. 81). Thus any air or blood in the chest cavity can drain out into the bottle and is easily recognised but air cannot be sucked back. One word of warning, however, is necessary. During transportation of the patient

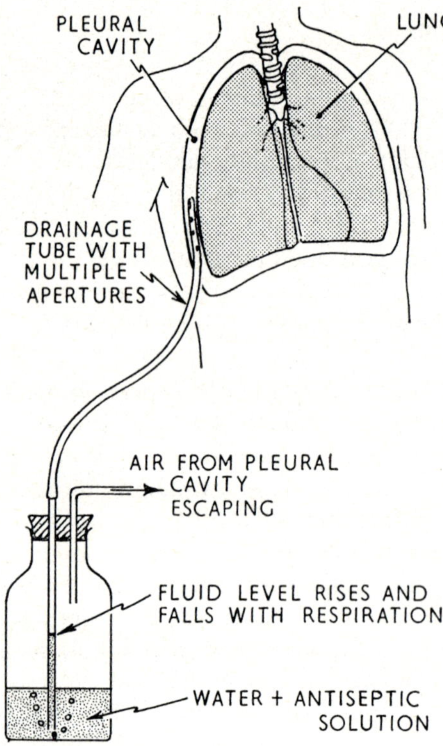

FIG. 81
Water-seal drain: It is important that the chest drain be attached to the glass tube which opens under the surface of the liquid in the bottle.

or moving him about in bed the under water seal must always be kept at a lower level than the chest, unless the tubing is clamped; otherwise the fluid in the bottle will flow back into the chest. If the chest drainage tube is patent the level of the fluid in the descending glass tube will fluctuate smoothly with respiration. If it does not, then the tube is probably blocked with debris or clotted blood and must be gently " milked " until patent again. Another method of ensuring safe drainage of the pleural cavity is by use of a one-way valve which prevents air entering the chest (Fig. 82).

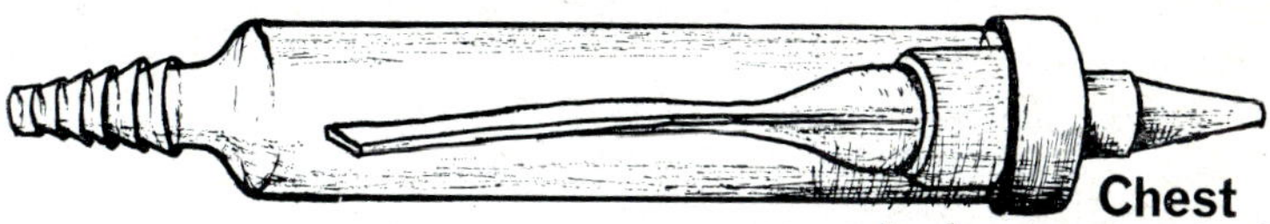

FIG. 82

The Heimlich Valve: This one-way valve is interposed between the chest drain and the drainage bottle. Air and blood may flow in the direction indicated but the rubber valve prevents air entering the pleural cavity.

After an intrathoracic operation patients may have a considerable amount of wound pain and pleural irritation from the drain. This discourages movement, deep breathing and coughing and results in retention of secretions in the bronchi, hypoxia and carbon dioxide retention. Suitable doses of analgesics must be given to permit adequate respiratory effort to be maintained and coughing must be encouraged to clear the airway of secretions. Nowhere is the value of the post-operative recovery room more apparent than in the care of these patients.

7. Post-craniotomy Patients

The intensive care of patients who have undergone neurosurgical procedures is worthy of special mention. These patients may be conscious or unconscious. In the case of the conscious patient the problem usually resolves itself into the careful observation of the conscious level, the cardiopulmonary state and the ensuring of adequate nutrition. Where the patient is unconscious, meticulous attention must be paid to alterations in the level of consciousness and for this purpose a special chart is of assistance (page 191). Signs of increased intracranial pressure are an indication for urgent intervention to avoid irreparable cerebral damage from " coning ". The measurement of central venous pressure is invaluable as an uncontrolled rise can result in increased intracranial pressure.

The management of the airway in those patients is as always of paramount importance since hypoxia or carbon dioxide retention can increase cerebral oedema and prejudice the patient's recovery. The use of naso-tracheal tubes is of great assistance here and reduces the need for tracheostomy. Active cooling measures may be required where hyperthermia is a complication.

INHALATION THERAPY

The gas most commonly utilised in inhalation therapy is oxygen, although mixtures of oxygen with carbon dioxide (in carbon monoxide poisoning) or helium (in respiratory obstruction) are occasionally used. Increasing the concentration of oxygen, even to 100 per cent., in the inspired gas or air is of limited value if respiratory obstruction or inadequate respiration is present. Where hypoxia is present and oxygen therapy instituted the person who orders this treatment must ensure that the airway is clear and ventilation adequate—or he should seek help. Delivering 100 per cent. oxygen to the face of an apnoeic patient without ensuring a clear airway and manually or mechanically assisting ventilation is futile.

Rationale of Oxygen Therapy

Ambient air contains approximately 21 per cent. oxygen at a partial pressure of about 150 mm. Hg (1/5 of 760 mm. Hg). When a patient breathes 100 per cent. oxygen the nitrogen in the lungs is " washed " out and the partial pressure of oxygen in the lungs is increased to nearly 760 mm. Hg. Thus the pressure gradient for oxygen diffusion across the alveolar capillary membrane is greatly increased, more oxygen is dissolved in the plasma and the plasma content is increased approximately sevenfold. It is apparent that any further increase in the plasma content of oxygen can only be achieved by raising the ambient pressure above normal. This is a technique which requires a pressure chamber and those in current use, raise the ambient pressure from 1 atmosphere (760 mm. Hg) to 2 and for some purposes 3 atmospheres. At 3 atmospheres the plasma content of oxygen is increased to 5·6 ml. 0_2/100 ml. plasma which is almost sufficient to maintain life without the oxygen linked to haemoglobin, since around 5 ml. 0_2/100 ml. blood is the basic metabolic requirement.

Toxic Effects of Oxygen Therapy

1. In patients with respiratory disease depending on " hypoxic drive " to the respiratory centre to maintain respiration, uncontrolled oxygen administration can lead to respiratory depression and even apnoea.

2. Prolonged oxygen therapy results in vasoconstriction and in neonates leads to retrolental fibroplasia if concentrations greater than 40 per cent. are administered.

3. Pulmonary damage with oedema may follow prolonged administration of 100 per cent. oxygen.

4. Prolonged exposure to 100 per cent. oxygen at raised ambient pressures (2-3 atmospheres) can cause disturbance to the central nervous system with convulsions. In addition severe pain in the air sinuses and middle ear may occur.

Methods of Administration

There are four main methods of oxygen administration.

1. *Nasal Catheter*: This method is of use where only a modest increase in the inspired oxygen concentration is desired. Low flows of about 3 litres/minute are well tolerated by the patient and this gives an inspired oxygen concentration of about 25 per cent.

2. *Masks*: Many differing types of mask are now available, plastic disposable ones being most popular. Higher flow rates are tolerated by the patient but the flow rate must never be less than the patient's minute volume or rebreathing and carbon dioxide retention will occur. The average adult requires a flow of at least 8 litres oxygen/minute which will give an inspired oxygen concentration of 50-60 per cent.

3. *Venturi Masks*. This type of mask, making use of the Venturi principle, enables the physician to control more accurately the oxygen concentration administered to the patient. Thus oxygen can be administered to patients with hypoxic drive with less risk of respiratory depression.

4. *The Edinburgh Mask* (Fig. 83). This simple disposable mask is also designed for the delivery of controlled *low concen-*

trations of oxygen to patients with hypoxic drive. A modification, the addition of a reservoir, enables the same mask to be used for the delivery of *high concentrations* of oxygen where required.

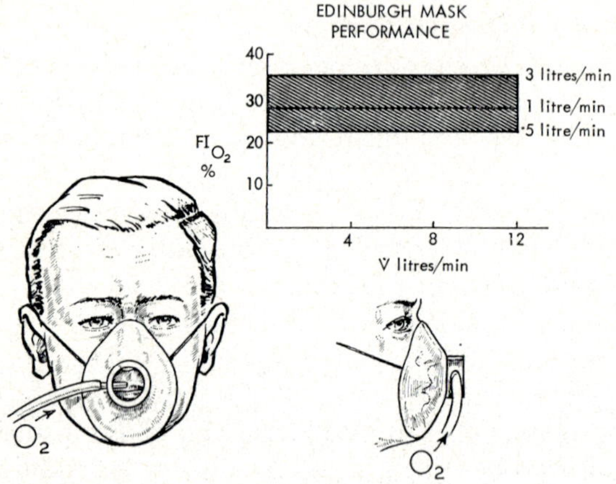

FIG. 83

The Edinburgh Mask. The inset graph shows the percentage of oxygen in the inspired gas mixture ($FI_{O_2}\%$) achieved by delivering different flow rates of oxygen to the open-ended mask. It can be seen that the percentage of oxygen breathed by the patient varies little with changes in the minute volume ($\dot{V}$ litres/minute). (After Flenley, D. C., Hutchison, D. C. S. & Donald, K. W. (1963). *Brit. med. J.* **2,** 1081.)

5. *Oxygen Tents*: This method is not now so popular as formerly. The tent makes nursing difficult and many patients become claustrophobic. Continual opening and closing of the tent to permit nursing procedures results in practice in low oxygen concentrations.

Oxygen as a Vehicle for Drug Administration: Bronchodilator drugs such as isoprenaline or orciprenaline can be administered in a fine droplet suspension in oxygen using a nebuliser attachment to the administration apparatus. This technique is useful in patients with bronchospasm particularly when combined with the inhalation of mucolytic agents such as chymotrypsin or "Alevaire," to liquefy the tenacious sputum. Antibiotics may also be administered in this way although it is more logical and efficient to give them by injection.

Control of Oxygen Therapy

It would quite reasonably be thought rash if a clinician were to administer a potent drug from an uncalibrated syringe. Oxygen is a widely used drug and its safe and effective administration requires similar control. Such control implies measurements of two kinds. Firstly, measurement of the dose administered to the patient and secondly, measurement of the effect of the drug on the patient's condition. The following are the various ways in which oxygen administration can be controlled.

1. *Methods of Measuring Amount of Oxygen Delivered*:

Flowmeter: This device measures in litres/minute the flow of oxygen delivered to the patient.

Oxygen Analyser: Different types of analyser are available for sampling the inspired concentration ($F_{I_{O_2}}$) breathed by the patient from mask or ventilator. This measurement should be made at the same time as the patient's arterial oxygen saturation and tension are measured in order to relate one to the other.

2. *Methods of Assessing Therapy in Patients*:

Colour of skin and mucosae: This is unreliable since hypoxaemia can exist in the absence of cyanosis. In addition, lighting conditions and the state of the patient's peripheral circulation can lead to erroneous assessment.

Oximetry: Apparatus is available which measures the arterial haemoglobin oxygen saturation indirectly by detecting the changes in light reflection through the patient's capillary bed e.g. in the ear-lobe. This method is imprecise where the peripheral circulation is poor.

Arterial Oxygen Measurement: This is the most accurate technique. An arterial blood sample is used and the percentage saturation of the haemoglobin with oxygen (Sa_{O_2}) and the arterial oxygen tension (Pa_{O_2}) estimated. To facilitate repeated measurements in acute illness, indwelling arterial cannulae may be employed.

SEDATIVES, ANALGESICS AND HYPNOTICS

The provision of "sedation" for patients under his care is one of the first tasks to face the house officer in hospital. By definition, to sedate means to soothe or settle, but it is customary to use the term sedative to describe drugs which relieve anxiety, while the terms analgesic and hypnotic are correctly applied to pain relieving and sleep producing agents respectively.

There is often an overlap in the actions of a drug, some analgesics, notably the opiates, relieving anxiety and many sedatives, for example the barbiturates, in larger doses inducing sleep. It is therefore essential in selecting the appropriate drug to decide whether the aim is to remedy pain, anxiety or restlessness. It must be remembered also that if a drug is prescribed within a few hours of the beginning or end of an operation it may interact with other drugs used during anaesthesia producing deeper or longer sleep than expected and/or more severe depression of blood pressure or respiration than is desirable. For the safety of the patient, the house officer and anaesthetist should co-operate in deciding what drugs are to be given immediately before and after operation.

Pain Relief

If pain is present an analgesic should be administered. For milder or more chronic pain one may use Tabs. Codein. Co. or Tabs. Paracetamol, one to two, orally, four hourly. Pain of greater severity may respond to dihydrocodeine bitartrate (DF 118) 30-60 mg. or pentazocine 50-75 mg. by mouth.

For severe pain, particularly in the post-operative period, the opiates or pethidine are still the drugs of choice. Morphine sulphate 10-15 mg., papaveretum 10-20 mg. or pethidine 50-100 mg. can be given parenterally for the average adult patient (70 Kg. body weight). Pentazocine 20-30 mgm. may also be used. Pentazocine is claimed to be a non-addicting analgesic and is related to the opiate antagonist nalorphine. Its duration of action is shorter than that of morphine but the incidence of emetic sequelae is also considerably lower. Both this drug and phenazocine which has addictive qualities may be used in combination with a non-analgesic sedative, e.g. promazine or promethazine. In this way the action of the drug is enhanced and prolonged, and emetic sequelae further reduced.

The combination of morphine and cyclizine (Cyclimorph) is also worth considering in patients who are experiencing severe pain but have severe nausea and vomiting when opiates are used to relieve the pain. In selecting *the correct dose* consideration should be given to the patient's physical state, his weight and any other drugs given recently. Many anaesthetists give the first post-operative dose of analgesic in dilute solution intravenously, e.g. morphine 10 mg., or pethidine 100 mg. in 10 ml. water, taking several minutes to complete the injection and stopping the injection when pain is relieved. This technique is best employed initially under supervision. The opiates provide better psychic sedation than pethidine and in equi-analgesic doses (morphine 10 mg.≡pethidine 60-65 mg.) there is little difference in side effects, i.e. respiratory depression and nausea and vomiting. Papaveretum is claimed to produce less respiratory depression and nausea than morphine because of the papaverine content but in equi-analgesic dosage with morphine the degree of respiratory and cardiovascular depression is similar. The respiratory depression produced by all three drugs may be antagonised by the intravenous injection of nalorphine 5-10 mg. or levallorphan 1-2 mg. Care must be taken not to overshoot the dose of these drugs necessary to reverse the respiratory depression present since the effect is then to increase the depression. The use of a pre-mixed combination of pethidine and levallorphan (100 mg.: 1·25 mg.) has little to recommend it except that it serves to remind all concerned that they are dealing with a patient who is liable to develop respiratory insufficiency. NEVER give barbiturates or phenothiazine drugs to a patient suffering severe pain unless an analgesic is given at the same time. These drugs increase the sensitivity of the patient to pain and cause marked restlessness. Remember also that in many patients post-operatively the peripheral circulation may be impaired and absorption of an opiate injected subcutaneously may be delayed. In these cases, and when using larger or irritant injections, intramuscular injection is indicated.

Relief of anxiety may help to relieve pain and the use of the benzodiazepines is of value. Bear in mind also the value of reassurance and attention to bodily comfort—keeping the patient warm for example. Also of immense value is some form of distraction such as conversation with other patients. Finally, for painful dressings premixed nitrous oxide and oxygen as used in labour (p. 206) may be employed. It may be used also to supplement narcotic therapy preceding and during physiotherapy.

The problem of recognising pain in patients on ventilators is discussed at page 183.

For the first few days after a major operation an opiate is usually indicated but thereafter night sedation may take the form of a hypnotic along with Tabs. Codein. Co. or Tabs. Paracetamol. The change should be made from the more potent drugs as soon as practicable to reduce the liability to addiction.

Anxiety

This is a common complaint in a hospital ward and one which is all too often ignored. The administration of phenobarbitone or amylobarbitone (30 mg. of either orally) thrice daily is valuable. The use of tranquillisers such as chlordiazepoxide is more expensive but may cause less drowsiness.

Insomnia

There is a large number of drugs available to induce sleep. Of the barbiturates pentobarbitone, quinalbarbitone, butobarbitone or amylobarbitone, 100-200 mg. orally are adequate for most purposes. In the elderly, the barbiturates, and in particular pentobarbitone, may cause restlessness and confusion and are better avoided. Glutethimide (Doriden) 250-500 mg. or methaqualone 150-300 mg. orally are useful alternatives.

Restlessness

Restlessness may be associated with pain in the patient recovering from anaesthesia but not yet fully conscious. This restlessness usually responds to an analgesic. In the conscious patient it may be associated with anxiety in which case it responds to a barbiturate or tranquilliser. RESTLESSNESS MAY BE ASSOCIATED WITH INADEQUATE RESPIRATION OR CONCEALED HAEMORRHAGE and these must be excluded as the injudicious use of sedatives may be lethal in such cases. In other cases restlessness is associated with head injury or is found in older patients. Promazine or chlorpromazine 25-50 mg. orally or intramuscularly is of value in some of these cases but a specialist opinion is usually desirable before treating a restless patient where the cause is not obvious.

Paraldehyde 10-15 ml. orally or rectally or up to 0·2 ml./Kg. intramuscularly should be reserved for otherwise uncontrollable patients.

In conclusion the following are important points to remember:

1. Always use a drug appropriate to the symptom being treated—analgesics for pain, hypnotics for insomnia, etc.
2. Learn to use a small number of effective drugs.
3. Remember the placebo effect. Forty per cent. of patients obtain pain relief from injections of saline, and many patients sleep after taking inert tablets. Your drugs must do better than this if they are to be effective.
4. When dealing with restless patients always look for and deal with the cause if possible. This may involve consulting a senior clinician.
5. Consider what other drugs the patient has had recently or what other drugs he is likely to receive during anaesthesia or in the post-operative period.
6. Keep a clear record of all drugs given, their dosage, route, time of administration and effect, where others will see the record before further drugs are prescribed.
7. Do not prescribe powerful drugs four or six hourly. Many are cumulative, and the need for further injection should be established.

CHAPTER XI

THE RESPIRATORY INTENSIVE CARE UNIT

The post-operative recovery phase usually lasts from one to twenty-four hours. However, certain patients may require much longer special care and they are best accommodated in an intensive care unit, where other patients, not necessarily post-operative, are intensively nursed for longer periods of time, e.g. two days to six weeks.

This pattern of progressive care of patients throughout their stay in hospital can be applied more widely than to surgical patients alone. Figure 84 demonstrates schematically the various

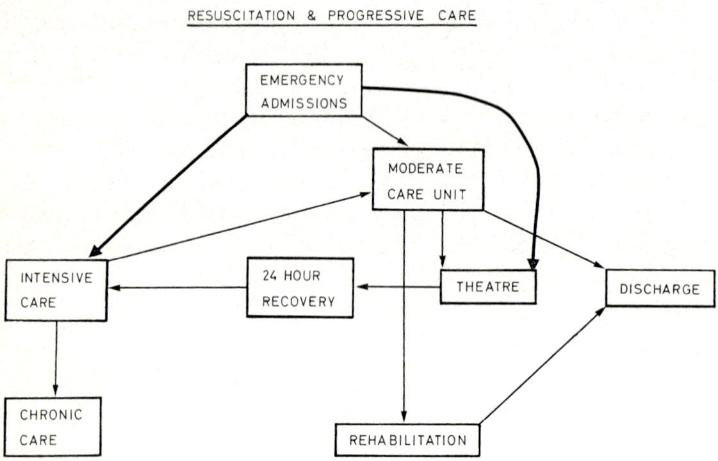

FIG. 84

pathways the patient may follow after reception at an emergency admission unit until his ultimate discharge from hospital. In any individual case the sole consideration which determines the patient's place of treatment is the degree of observation and the amount of therapy required. The most ill patients are, therefore, gathered together in areas where staff and equipment are concentrated to enable intensive observation and therapy to be undertaken. Intensive care areas are made up of individual units restricted to the treatment of a particular group of patients, e.g. respiratory emergencies, artificial kidney cases, acute coronary occlusion cases (Fig. 85).

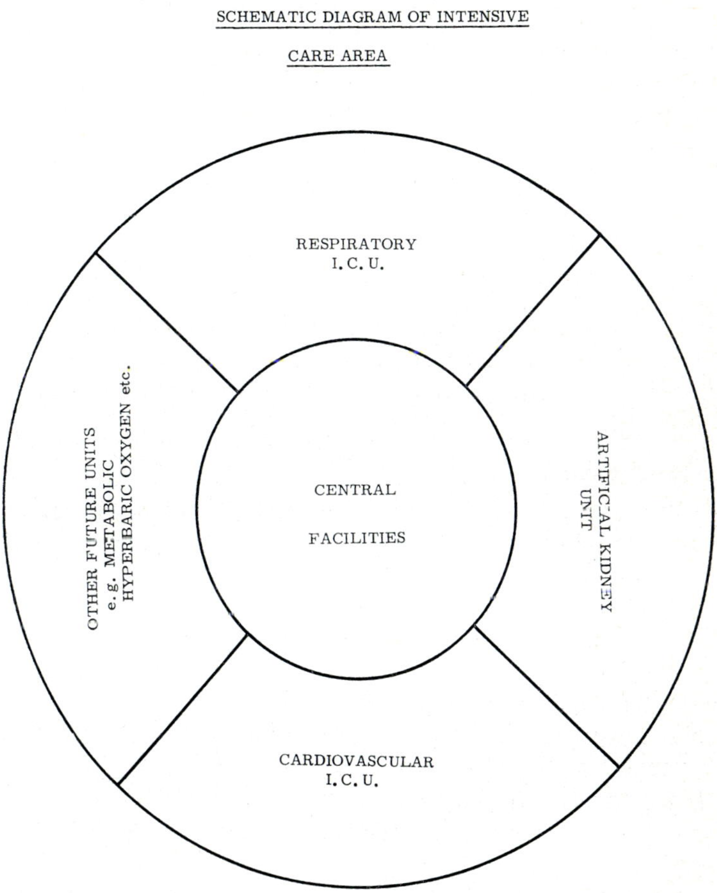

FIG. 85

The anaesthetist is mainly concerned with that part of the intensive care area where patients with respiratory problems are treated, and it is this type of patient whom we shall consider here. The following are some of the conditions which can lead to a patient's admission to the Respiratory Intensive Care Unit.

1. Post-operative respiratory insufficiency.
2. Severe head injuries and facio-maxillary injuries.
3. Trauma to the chest wall: crushed-chest injuries.
4. Obstructive lung disease with respiratory failure (emphysema with an additional acute respiratory infection).
5. Carbon monoxide and barbiturate poisoning.
6. Certain infectious diseases: poliomyelitis, polyneuritis, tetanus.
7. Miscellaneous medical conditions: cerebrovascular accidents, myasthenia gravis, acute porphyria.

SPECIAL PROCEDURES IN THE RESPIRATORY UNIT

The methods and manoeuvres used in the recovery room are, of course, also practised in the respiratory unit, but a knowledge of some additional procedures is essential.

1. Tracheostomy

If assistance to ventilation is required it is usually necessary to do this with a cuffed endotracheal tube in place (see page 106). This enables secretions in the bronchi to be aspirated and usually ensures an unobstructed airway. The tracheal tube is a temporary expedient and is not commonly left in place beyond 24-48 hours. For longer periods of treatment an uncuffed nasotracheal tube may be used particularly in children. Where this type of assistance is required for an indefinite period it is usual to perform a tracheostomy.

INDICATIONS. Although the operation is performed for many varying surgical and medical conditions these fall readily into two main groups:—

(*a*) Conditions in which there is obstruction to the patient's airway, particularly in its upper part, e.g. acute oedema of the glottis and carcinoma of larynx. The value of tracheostomy is obvious here—the obstruction is bypassed and free and tranquil respiration ensues.

(*b*) The second group of conditions, where tracheostomy is indicated, is the one in which impairment of the patient's respiratory function, other than simple airway obstruction, is a threat to life. The causes of respiratory insufficiency

(Chap. IX) have been already dealt with and may vary from acute trauma to poliomyelitis. Usually such patients have no cough or, at best, an ineffective one and secretions rapidly accumulate in the airway and must be removed.

ADVANTAGES OF TRACHEOSTOMY

1. Reduction of the respiratory "dead space" by approximately half. Each breath is now used more effectively to

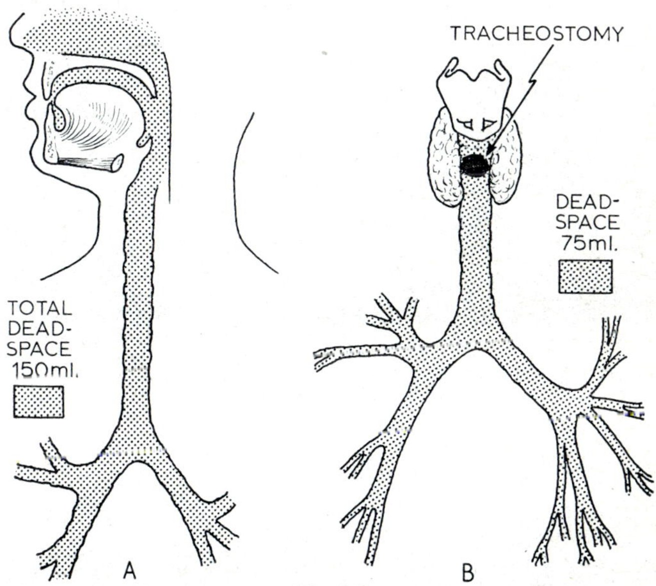

FIG. 86

The stippled area represents the volume of the "dead-space" gases which take no part in respiration. A shows the volume of dead-space in the normal adult while B illustrates the considerable reduction effected by tracheostomy. For the same respiratory effort an extra 75 ml. of air is now drawn into the depths of the lungs and is thus available for gas-exchange.

oxygenate the blood and remove carbon dioxide from it (Fig. 86).

2. Easier removal of secretions from the air passages.

3. A reduction in the work of respiration and in oxygen requirements results from 1 and 2.

4. Better control of oxygen administration is possible via a tracheostomy box and humidifier (Fig. 87).

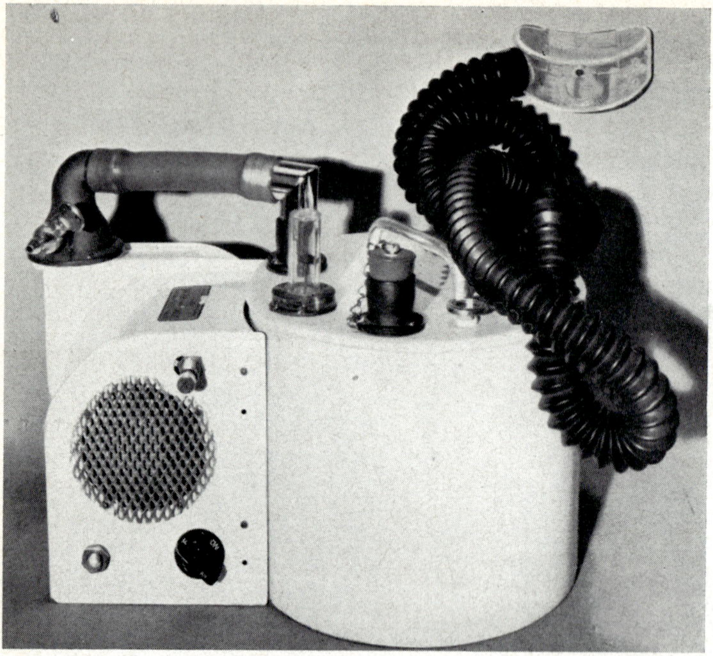

Fig. 87

The perspex tracheostomy box is shown in the right upper portion of the photograph, in this case connected by the corrugated tubing to a humidifier.

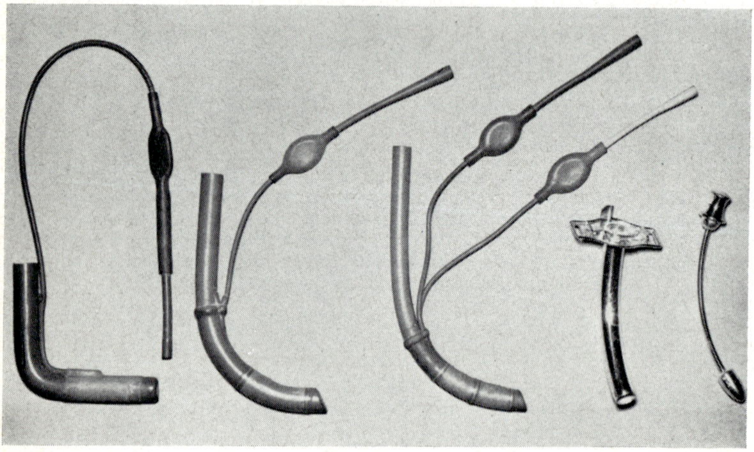

Fig. 88

Tracheostomy tubes: four types of tube in common use are shown (from left to right), the James, the Rüsch, the double-cuffed Rüsch and the standard silver tube.

5. In patients with depressed pharyngeal and laryngeal reflexes, e.g. cough reflex and swallowing, the lungs can be sealed off from the danger of aspirated secretions and gastric contents, by the use of a cuffed tracheostomy tube (Fig. 88).

6. Should mechanical assistance to ventilation be required in addition, this is facilitated by a tracheostomy.

MANAGEMENT OF TRACHEOSTOMY. In order that the patient may benefit fully from this procedure certain problems of management must be understood and overcome.

(*a*) *Care of Tubes*: It is customary to insert a tube through the tracheostomy opening into the trachea. The familiar double-silver tube is still used, but usually when the patient is on the way to recovery. In the early stages, however, one of the cuffed variety is preferred as this type of tube provides an effective seal for the lungs against secretions and makes possible assisted or controlled ventilation, should this be required. Over-inflation of the cuff for long periods can lead to excessive pressure on the tracheal mucosa and to necrosis and sloughing. This can be avoided by inflation of the cuff to make a seal without excessive pressure and, by deflation of the cuff at intervals, for a short time. Deflation of the cuff must always be preceded by thorough oropharyngeal suction so that secretions will not run down alongside the tube into the lungs. A new type of double-cuffed tube (the Rüsch tube) further reduces these hazards in that the two cuffs can be alternately deflated and inflated, to reduce the chances of mucosal ulceration but, at no time, are the lungs entirely without protection. Tubes must be changed frequently particularly when the sputum is copious and viscid since the inside becomes encrusted with dried secretions. Otherwise the lumen of the tube gradually becomes blocked and death from acute asphyxia may result. Tracheostomy tubes are usually changed at least every 48 hours.

After use, the tube must be cleaned and autoclaved, before being used again. The use of disposable plastic tubes, both single and double-cuffed, obviates many of the difficulties of cleansing and re-sterilising of rubber tubes (Fig. 89).

(*b*) *Humidification*: Since the paranasal sinuses and nasopharynx, whose function is to warm and humidify the inspired air, have been bypassed by the tracheostomy, it is necessary to provide an alternative source of moisture and heat, to avoid hardening of the secretions and drying and fissuring of the mucosa of the respiratory tract. This can be done in various ways:—

(*i*) It may be sufficient to inject small quantities (e.g. 0·5 ml.) of sterile saline down the tracheostomy tube at intervals.

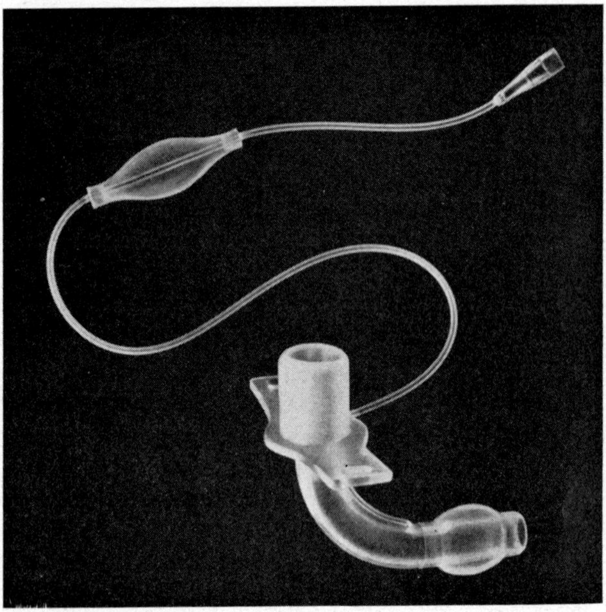

FIG. 89
The Portex Disposable Tracheostomy Tube.

(*ii*) If the patient is breathing room air, then, in a humid climate, it is often sufficient to conserve the moisture in the patient's own expirations with a simple condenser humidifier (Fig. 90). The moisture in each expiration condenses on the wire-mesh and revaporises on inspiration. Condenser humidifiers are efficient only when the mesh remains reasonably dry and so it must be changed repeatedly, usually three hourly, and dried. The wire-mesh serves also to trap large dust particles and prevent their inhalation.

(*iii*) In a dry climate, where the atmosphere contains little water vapour, or when the patient breathes oxygen, which is delivered free of moisture and fairly cold from the cylinder or pipe-line, active warming and humidification is usually required. This is done by passing the oxygen or air/oxygen

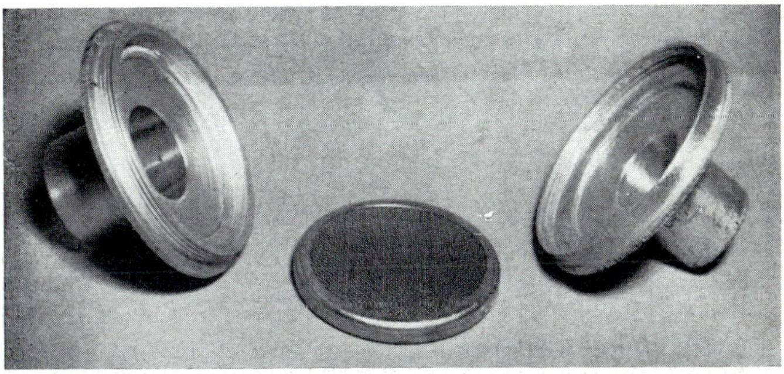

FIG. 90
The Condenser Humidifier: the two parts of the humidifier have been unscrewed to reveal the removable wire-gauze insert.

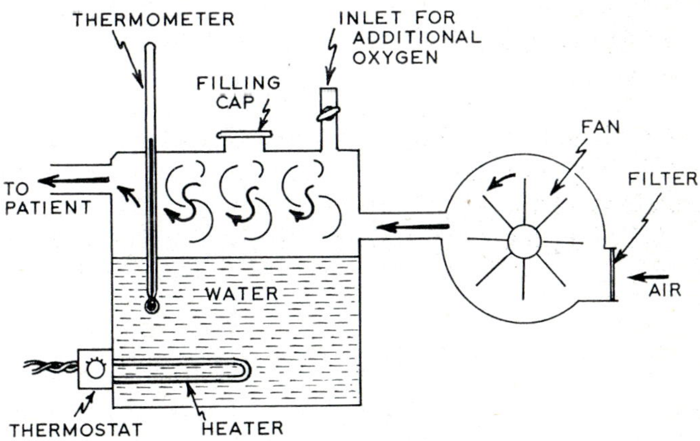

FIG. 91
The Tank Humidifier: Air or air and oxygen are blown over the surface of the warm water and then to the patient.

mixture through a " tank " type humidifier (Fig. 91) which warms the gas to about body temperature and saturates it with water-vapour. The warm and moist oxygen then passes along a tube to a perspex tracheostomy box (Fig. 87) mounted over the tracheostomy tube. This box has a series of holes in its surface to permit free expiration and elimination of carbon dioxide, which would otherwise accumulate. There is also a port-hole, with a cover which slides to one side, to give access for tracheal suction.

(*iv*) Other devices designed to solve the problem of humidification act like perfume " atomisers " and propel a fine spray of water droplets into the stream of air or oxygen as it is inspired. These devices have the advantage that bronchodilator drugs, e.g. isoprenaline (Neo-Epinine) or antibiotics may be suspended in the water and delivered into the depths of the lungs.

Before leaving the subject of humidification it is necessary to mention, if only to condemn, the practice of " humidifying " oxygen by bubbling it through a Wolff's bottle. This device is not an efficient method of adding moisture to the inspired gases.

(*c*) *Endobronchial Suction*: The care with which secretions are aspirated from the patient's airway is of the greatest importance. The accent should always be on sterility, thoroughness and gentleness.

It is obvious that the patient is at risk from whatever lethal organism is carelessly introduced due to inadequate sterile technique. If not of the disposable type the endobronchial catheters should be used only once and then cleaned and autoclaved. The catheter used for oropharyngeal suction should not be used for suction through the tracheostomy. The hands should be scrubbed before each period of suction and should never come in contact with that portion of the catheter which enters the patient's airway.

Tracheal suction should be carried out as often as is necessary to keep the airways free from secretions. The more copious the secretions, the more often must the manoeuvre be repeated. Whenever possible two people should co-operate during this time, one carrying out the aspiration and the other turning the patient from one side to the other to ensure that the catheter enters both right and left main bronchi.

The calibre of the catheter selected is important. Its diameter should be less than half that of the tracheostomy tube, otherwise it will partially or completely block it and cause acute asphyxia. The catheter should be " nipped " between finger and thumb when introduced and released to allow suction only on withdrawal, otherwise there is a real danger that excessive suction will collapse portions of the lung. The negative pressure should never be greater than is required to remove the secretions easily. More powerful suction is required when the sputum is thick and tenacious. At all times, the catheter should be handled gently to avoid unnecessary trauma to the sensitive mucosa of the respiratory tract.

Complications of Tracheostomy

1. *Infection*: Tracheostomy opens up a route for secondary infection of the lungs and hence the management of such cases must be attended by scrupulous aseptic precautions.

2. *Loss of humidification*: Loss of the normal humidification of the inspired gases by the paranasal sinuses and nasopharynx results in crusting of secretions in the airway.

3. *Mucosal ulceration*: Due to excessive pressure in the tracheostomy tube cuff.

4. *Dilatation of the trachea*: Overinflation of the tube cuff can, on occasion, result in erosion of the cartilaginous rings of the trachea and resultant dilatation.

5. *Granuloma*: Trauma to the tracheal mucosa can lead to the development of granulation tissue and a small polyp may result.

6. *Fistula formation*: This is a serious complication which may rarely occur. Excessive cuff pressure and other trauma lead to the formation of a tracheo-oesophageal fistula. Food and secretions enter the trachea below the cuff of the tube and contaminate the lungs.

7. *Sinus formation*: Imperfect healing of the post-tracheostomy stoma can result in a persistent sinus requiring surgical closure.

8. *Erosion of blood vessels*: Particularly if the stoma becomes infected, a blood vessel may be eroded by the tracheostomy tube and give rise to severe haemorrhage.

9. *Tracheal stricture*: In some 2 per cent. of patients with tracheostomy, who have had ventilator treatment, a stricture may develop either at the site of the cuff or at the lower end of the tube. This is a serious late complication often requiring difficult plastic surgery. It is commoner in young children

where the cross-section of the airway is quite small. Naso-tracheal intubation is preferred to tracheostomy in children to avoid this.

2. Mechanical Assistance to Ventilation (Intermittent Positive Pressure Ventilation: I.P.P.V.)

Before embarking on a description of mechanical assistance to ventilation it is necessary to consider some physiological aspects of the technique. Controlled ventilation, whether performed manually or mechanically, has certain potentially harmful effects on the respiratory and cardiovascular systems. Excessive pressures applied to the patient's airway may result in damage to lung tissue and even to rupture of the lungs. It is generally accepted that pressures exceeding +30 cm. H_2O at the mouth should be avoided and most machines in use incorporate a safety valve which automatically opens when the airway pressure exceeds this figure. In addition a pressure gauge is attached to the ventilator which gives a continuous reading of the pressure at the ventilator outlet and in some cases at the attachment to the patient's airway. The volume of gases entering and leaving the lungs is recorded on a spirometer or is pre-set by adjusting a control on the machine. Thus continuous observations of the stroke volume and cycling pressure of the ventilator and the frequency of ventilation can be made by the anaesthetist. The patient's ventilation requirements are predicted pre-operatively from such factors as body weight, sex, etc. (Fig. 29) and the ventilator can be adjusted to meet these requirements. Where equipment is available, blood gas analysis can be carried out at intervals to ensure adequate oxygenation and adequate elimination of carbon dioxide.

The potentially harmful effects of intermittent positive pressure ventilation on the cardiovascular system can result in a reduction in cardiac output and lead to cardiac failure. The explanation of this is to be found when we compare the intrathoracic pressure changes which accompany spontaneous respiration with those occurring during controlled ventilation (Fig. 92). It can be seen that normally the intrapulmonary and intrapleural pressures are negative during inspiration and in fact this assists the venous return to the right side of the heart—the " thoracic pump " mechanism. During expiration, the intrapulmonary pressure is positive and the intrapleural pressure is still negative although reduced. When controlled ventilation is employed these intrathoracic pressures are reversed and there is some interference with central venous return and obstruction to the pulmonary blood flow. The normal individual is able to compensate for these effects but in severely ill or shocked patients they can result in a reduction in cardiac output and hypotension.

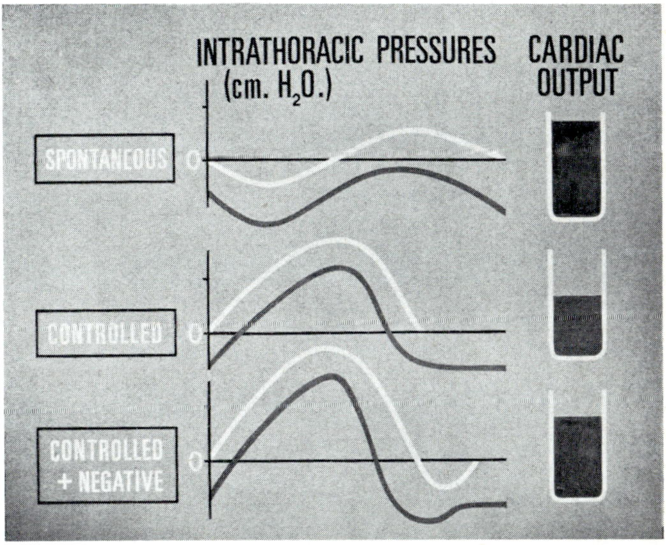

FIG. 92

A diagrammatic representation of the effect of various respiratory patterns on the cardiac output. The white line represents the intrapulmonary or alveolar pressure and the black line the intrapleural pressure. The addition of a negative phase, during mechanically controlled ventilation, compensates to some extent for the potentially harmful effect of this technique on cardiac output.

The use of a negative phase during the expiratory cycle of the ventilator will minimise this cardiovascular disturbance. This negative pressure should not exceed -5 cm. H_2O or it may lead to collapse of diseased bronchioles in patients with chronic respiratory disease.

In patients in whom respiratory inadequacy is severe or in whom there is no spontaneous respiration it is necessary to ventilate the lungs, either manually or with a mechanical ventilator. The manual method, using a device such as the Ambu resuscitator, is convenient in emergencies and for short periods of time. For prolonged ventilation recourse must be had to ventilators or respirators. It is important to avoid using the terms " ventilator " and " respirator " as if they are synonymous. Ventilators produce rhythmic inflation and deflation of the patient's lungs by intermittently delivering gases at a pressure above atmospheric pressure by way of a face-mask, endotracheal tube or tracheostomy tube (Fig. 93).

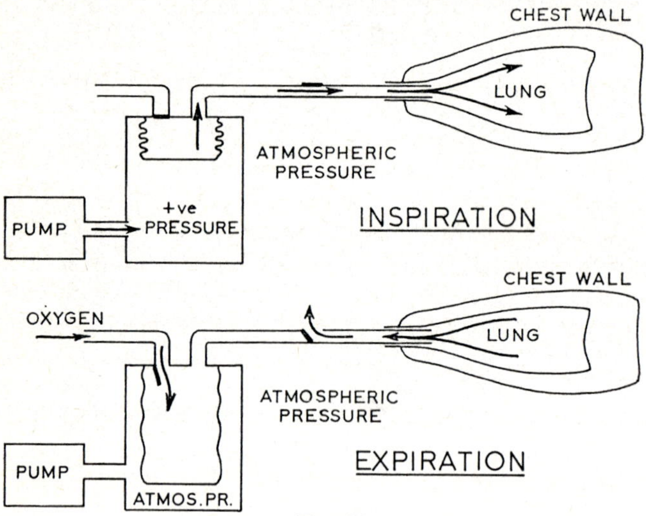

FIG. 93

Diagram of Ventilator Action: The bellows or bag containing the fresh gases is enclosed in an airtight chamber and squeezed during inspiration by the action of a pump which raises the pressure inside the chamber above the outside or atmospheric pressure. Thus the fresh gases are propelled into the patient's lungs through the endotracheal tube. During expiration, the pressure in the chamber falls again to atmospheric and the stale gases flow out of the lungs escaping to the outside air through a valve. At the same time, the bellows fill with fresh gas in readiness for the next inspiration.

In a sense, they act as another pair of hands, squeezing the bellows for the anaesthetist. Respirators, on the other hand, produce inflation and deflation of the patient's lungs by applying intermittent suction to the patient's chest-wall from the outside (Fig. 94).

Ventilators are preferred to respirators in most respiratory units since they permit better access to the patient for nursing needs and physiotherapy. The gases delivered from the ventilator are passed through a tank-humidifier on the way to the patient, since humidification is very important.

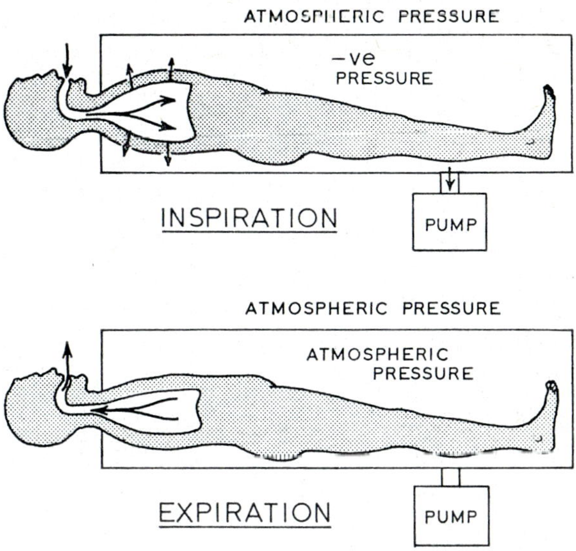

FIG. 94

Diagram of Respirator Action: The patient is entirely enclosed in an airtight box or tank (Tank Respirator) or sometimes the chest alone is enclosed (Cuirass Respirator). The pump's sucking action lowers the pressure within the box below the atmospheric pressure (−ve pressure) and the chest wall expands and the lungs fill with fresh gas or air during inspiration. Expiration occurs when the pump stops sucking and the pressure inside the box rises again to equal that of the surrounding air, the chest wall and lungs thus being allowed to return to their original position.

Management of Ventilator Cases

The successful management of ventilator cases requires the highest standards of skill and care. Figure 95 summarises some of the most important aspects of this treatment.

ROUTINE TRACHEOSTOMY RÉGIME: The routine care as for other tracheostomy cases is carried out but with one important modification. Most of the patients on ventilators are not breathing at all and can therefore only be disconnected for

FIG. 95

MANAGEMENT OF VENTILATOR CASE

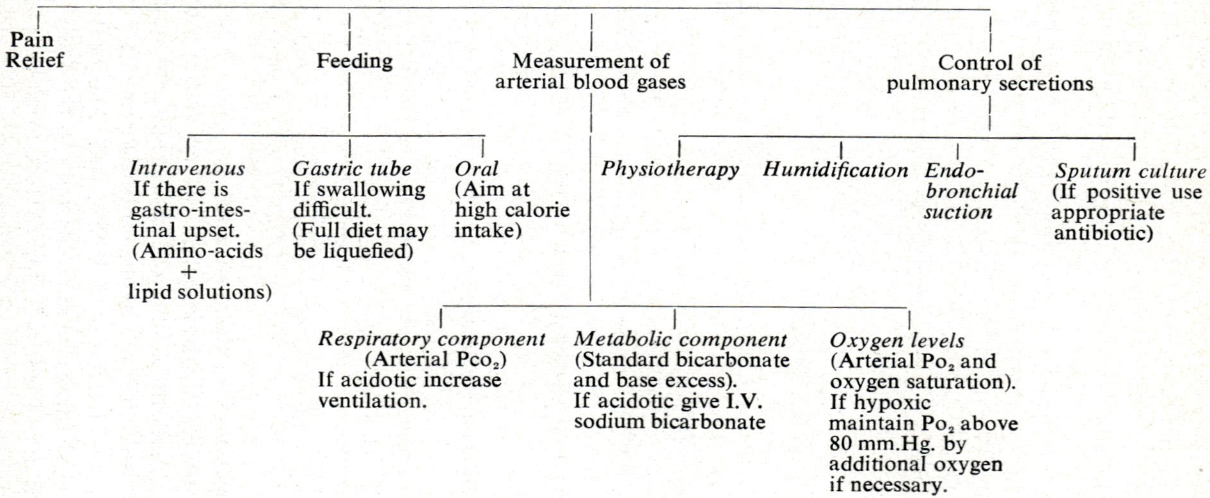

very short periods (approximately one minute) at a time to permit endobronchial suction. It is usually necessary to perform each period of suction in stages, allowing the patient a few " breaths " on the machine between each stage.

THE MANAGEMENT OF PAIN: During ventilator therapy the provision of adequate pain relief can present difficulties, especially in the patient who is unable to communicate. Although the available drugs and techniques of pain relief are many and varied, they are of little value in a situation where the clinician is unable to detect a need for them.

The patient normally reacts to unmodified pain in three possible ways:

(*a*) by making avoidance movements, i.e. attempting to withdraw the injured portion of the body from the stimulus.

(*b*) by responding autonomically, e.g. by changes in heart rate and systolic blood pressure,

(*c*) by responding at a cortical level in perceiving the ' painful ' stimulus and evaluating it against previous similar experience

Many of the patients on I.P.P.V. are incapable of the first response and indeed may be curarised. Although it has been claimed that the clinician can detect the higher response by complicated electroencephalographic techniques, this is impractical clinically. Measurements of the autonomic response are as yet the only practicable approach in this difficult situation.

The important thing for the clinician to remember is that an immobile, apparently tranquil, patient on I.P.P.V. may be suffering from considerable pain and its relief is an urgent matter. The method and drugs chosen will vary with the individual circumstances but the following list indicates the possibilities:

(*a*) *Parenteral analgesia.* Generally speaking, the intravenous route is to be preferred in this situation since the timing of the peak effect can be more certain and also the relief of pain achieved more quickly. Small incremental doses of say 2 mg. morphine sulphate are given intravenously until relief is obtained.

(*b*) *Inhalational analgesia.* It is technically simple with apparatus now available to administer inhalational agents to the patient receiving ventilator therapy. Volatile agents such as trichloroethylene and methoxyflurane can be given from accurately calibrated vaporisers in a 50:50 mixture of nitrous oxide in oxygen.

(*c*) *Regional blockade.* Where it is possible to induce a regional block, complete analgesia of the affected part without any risk of central depression can be achieved. The treatment can be repeated at intervals or maintained continuously as in the case of an epidural block.

GENERAL CARE AND PHYSIOTHERAPY: These patients must receive particular attention to pressure areas, oral hygiene, eyes and nose. The use of a " ripple-mattress " greatly reduces the chance of bed-sores developing. Many will have indwelling urinary catheters on continuous drainage and intravenous infusions which need constant attention. Passive maintenance exercises to the limbs, percussion of the chest wall and postural drainage are carried out regularly and the physiotherapist has an important function in the treatment of these patients.

NUTRITION: When a patient's illness is not severe or is of short duration inadequate nutrition may not lead to serious consequences. In traumatised patients who are receiving an inadequate calorie intake, the amount of tissue protein breakdown and nitrogen lost may be two to three times that in straightforward starvation. For every 10 grams of nitrogen excreted in the urine approximately 300 grams of muscle protein is lost and this process of catabolism is roughly proportional to the severity of surgery or trauma and is aggravated by the presence of sepsis. The patient in an intensive care unit who is gravely ill and in whom sepsis and abnormal electrolyte loss is present requires the most careful dietary care if a protracted stay in the unit or indeed a fatal outcome is to be avoided. In the past the metabolic response to severe illness or gross trauma was thought to be unavoidable. It is now known that the negative nitrogen balance which is a feature in these patients is largely reversible if food over and above the patient's normal requirement is provided.

The route of choice is by mouth if the patient is able to swallow and if there is no gastro-intestinal upset. If the patient cannot swallow then the patient can be tube fed. Where there is a gastro-intestinal upset such as paralytic ileus following surgery or injury it is possible to provide an adequate dietary intake intravenously employing amino acid solutions along with concentrated sugar solutions or fat emulsions as a source of calories. As the patient recovers, feeding by way of a nasal gastric tube will take the place of the intravenous infusions. The feeds are given in small bulk of high caloric value and with additional vitamin supplements, e.g. Complan. When the patient is able to swallow satisfactorily, oral feeding with a soft liquid diet is instituted. The dietitian's advice on nutritional problems can be invaluable at this stage and hasten the recovery process.

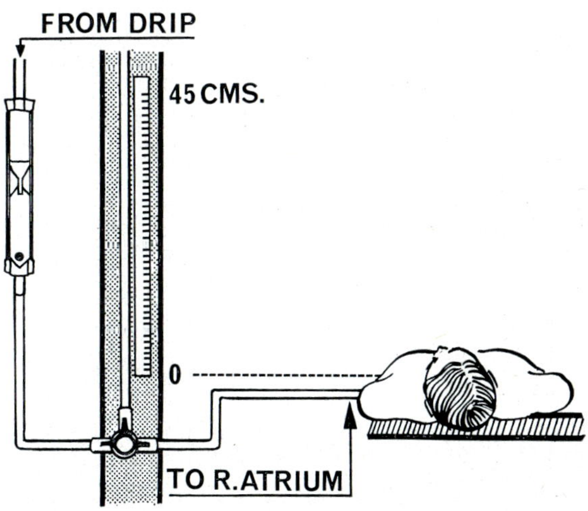

FIG. 96

Venous pressure manometer. A catheter is passed through the external jugular vein and into the right atrium and connected to a saline drip. The measuring column is connected to this system by a three-way tap. The zero on the centimetre scale must be level with the right atrium whenever a reading is being made—the mid-axillary line when the patient is lying down or the angle of the sternum when he is sitting up.

RECORDING OF VITAL FUNCTIONS: In addition to the regular recording of blood pressure, central venous pressure (Fig. 96), pulse rate and temperature, it is very important that the nurse, under the direction of the anaesthetist, should

Time and Date	O_2 Sat. or Po_2	pH	Pco_2	Stand. Bicarb.	Base Excess	Buffer Base	On Ventilator			Off Ventilator		Air Entry in Lungs		Remarks
							f	V_T	P	f	V_T	Left	Right	

FIG. 97

Ventilation Chart: Key to Symbols

O_2 saturation (O_2 sat.): the percentage of haemoglobin saturated with oxygen in the arterial blood.
Po_2: tension of oxygen in arterial blood.
pH: the degree of acidity or alkalinity of the blood in pH units.
Pco_2: the tension of carbon dioxide in the arterial blood. This is high in respiratory failure.

Standard bicarbonate, Base excess, Buffer base } These measurements indicate the efficiency of respiration and the body metabolism.

f: respiratory rate.
V_T: tidal volume.

P: the ventilator pressure during ventilation.
Air entry into lungs: A + or − in this column indicates the nurse's assessment of the degree of lung inflation using a stethoscope.

closely observe and record certain aspects of the ventilator's performance during treatment (Fig. 97). For each patient under treatment an ideal pattern of ventilation will have been chosen with regard to frequency of respiration, airway pressure (i.e. the pressure at the patient's mouth during each respiratory cycle of the machine) and the volume of gas being delivered to the patient's lungs (Fig. 98). Most respiratory units

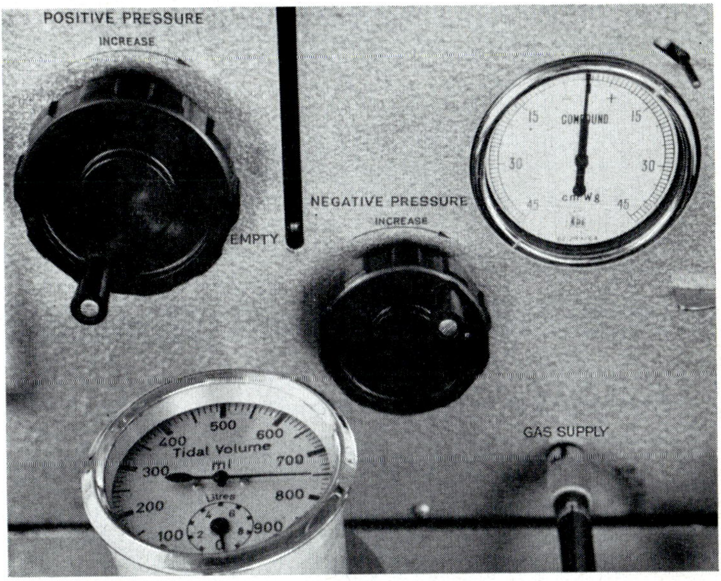

FIG. 98

The Drager respirometer attached to a ventilator can be seen in the left lower corner of the illustration. The gauge on the right measures the pressure required to inflate the patient's lungs.

have a chart on which these events, together with other relevant data, are recorded. The nurse is also trained to listen with a stethoscope over both lungs, at intervals, to make sure that the gases are entering the lungs and not being prevented from doing so by secretions in the upper airway or an obstructed tracheostomy tube.

During the intervals when the patient is disconnected from the ventilator to assess his ability to breathe spontaneously the nurse may be asked to make measurements of the tidal volume as well as the frequency of respiration. For this purpose a spirometer such as the Wright's model can be employed (Fig. 100).

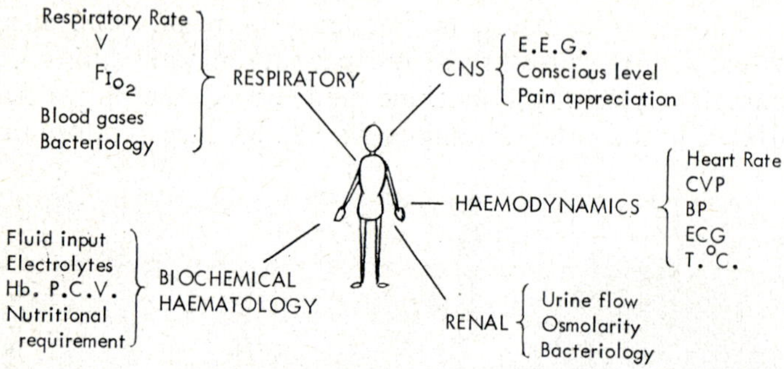

FIG. 99

Schematic diagram demonstrating the wide range of measurements required to guide the clinician in the management of a gravely ill patient in an intensive care unit.

Information about the patient's arterial blood gas levels (oxygen saturation, PO_2, pH, P_{CO_2} and standard bicarbonate), during intermittent positive pressure ventilation, is usually recorded on the ventilation chart by the anaesthetist and the pattern of ventilation may have to be changed at intervals to keep these levels as near normal as possible. The maintenance of electrolyte and water balance can be difficult in such cases and it is of the first importance to keep *accurate* records on a suitable *Input-Output* Chart. The hourly measurement of urine volume may be necessary in the most severely ill and renal function further assessed by regular measurement of urine and plasma osmolality.

MONITORING. It must be apparent that the type and number of observations to be made by the attending nurse, particularly on ventilator patients, are liable to be very time consuming (Fig. 99). In order to permit more frequent measurements to be made and to free the nurse for other important duties use is increasingly being made of centralised monitoring systems which en-enable one nurse to supervise a number of patients from the nursing station (Fig. 101). These systems can be designed to record temperature, heart rate, blood pressure and respiratory rate and indeed, in some very modern units, are combined with closed circuit television for each bed-station.

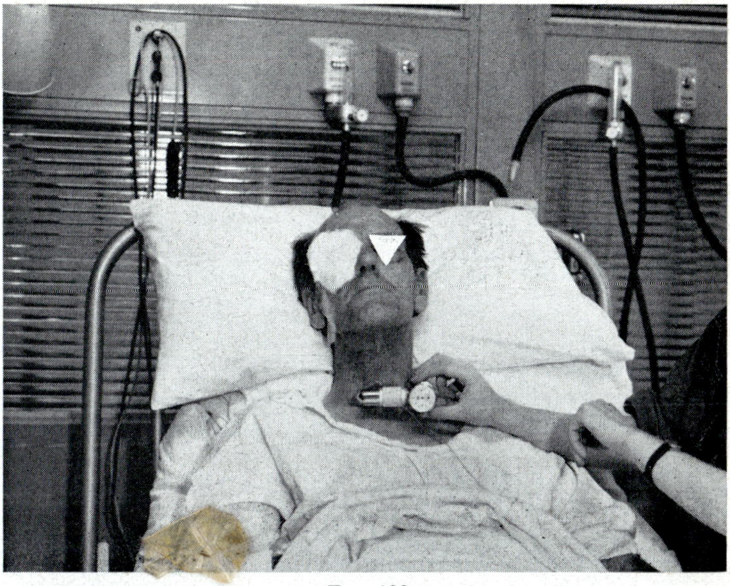

FIG. 100
The Wright's respirometer being used to measure a patient's minute volume. The instrument is shown attached to a tracheostomy tube.

THE CONTROL OF INFECTION. The operation of tracheostomy has been described as potentially lethal in that it opens up a direct route for infection to enter the patient's lungs. In addition, all the patients in an intensive care unit are severely ill and prone to intercurrent infection and it is therefore of the utmost importance to minimise the risk of cross-infection from one patient to the other and to isolate any cases of known infection by barrier nursing. Bed-stations should be at least 12 to 14 feet apart since this measure alone greatly reduces the risk of cross-infection. To facilitate isolation of infected cases cubicles are essential, preferably with separate entrances and exits.

A further measure which is of considerable assistance is to ventilate intensive care units, in the same manner as operating theatres, with filtered air from a positive pressure plenum system. Additional filters can be fitted to suction pumps and ventilator air-pumps to further safeguard the patients. All staff working in the unit should observe the accepted rules governing dress and conduct pertaining in operating theatres.

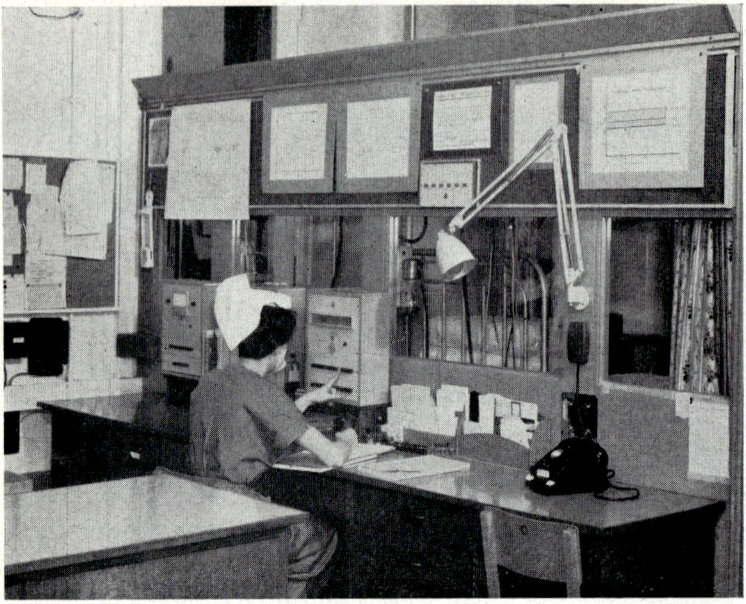

FIG. 101
The Nursing Station in the Respiratory Intensive Care Unit at Glasgow Royal Infirmary.

Staff-Patient Relationships: Many patients on I.P.P.V. are fully conscious but because of the tracheostomy cannot make their wants known to the nurse or doctor in the usual way. Often they become acutely depressed and despite continuing physical improvement lose their will to fight. The presence of understanding and cheerful staff can go a long way towards mitigating what is, for most, a strange and terrifying experience. Some may be able to write their requests and should always have a pad of paper and pencil at hand, but for others it is necessary to provide a large alphabet on which the patient can spell out a message with a finger. Great patience is required at this stage and one must be prepared to spend a lot of time in keeping up the patient's morale.

THE UNCONSCIOUS PATIENT

A varying proportion of the patients in the respiratory intensive care area are unconscious. Some of these may have head injuries alone or along with other injuries. Recording the level of unconsciousness is important and may be difficult. Accurate observations recorded frequently can be invaluable in assessing

Stage I	*II*	*III*	*IV*
Patient can answer simple questions	Patient can obey simple commands	Patient reacts only to painful stimuli	Patient fully unconscious. Does not react to any stimulus

FIG. 102

Date and Time	*Respiration*			*Pulse*		*Eyes*		*Muscle Tone*	*Reaction to Stimuli*	B.P.	*Estimated Level of Uncon-sciousness*
	Character	Depth	Rate	Volume	Rate	Pupil Size	React. to Light	Spastic or Flaccid	Question Commands Touch Pain		

FIG. 103

whether improvement or deterioration is taking place. The levels of consciousness may be classified as in Figure 102.

Other observations helpful in assessing these patients are rate, depth and character of respiration, rate and volume of pulse, blood pressure, central venous pressure, size of pupils and their reaction to light, muscle tone and presence of twitching or tremor and reaction to stimuli.

It is best if changes in all these observations are recorded; a chart (Fig. 103) eminently suitable for the purpose is that used in the Lambeth Hospital.*

* Broome, W. E. (1963). *Nurs. Mirror,* **115,** 415.

CHAPTER XII

RESUSCITATION

A. EXPIRED AIR RESUSCITATION OR MOUTH-TO-MOUTH BREATHING

History

Probably the first written account of this ancient technique is to be found in the Old Testament in the Second Book of Kings. There, a description is given of the "resuscitation" of a young boy by the prophet Elisha and for many hundreds

Physiology. Table of Constituents of Air Samples
(approximate values)

Gas	Atmospheric Air %	Alveolar Air %	Expired Air %
Oxygen	21	14·5	14 - 18
Carbon dioxide	0·04	5·5	4·5
Nitrogen and water vapour	79	80	79

FIG. 104

of years the method was known as "Elisha breathing". In 1954 Elam and his colleagues demonstrated that expired air resuscitation was more effective than the standard methods of "artificial respiration", e.g. Holger-Nielson and Schafer methods. In 1958 Safar described an airway he designed to make the method easier to perform and in 1960 the Brook airway was first produced.

It will be noted from Figure 104 that atmospheric air contains about 21 per cent. oxygen and minimal carbon dioxide. Provided an adequate amount of air is propelled into the depths of the lungs by the bellows action of the chest and diaphragm, and the airway is clear, the blood flowing through the lungs in the capillaries will be sufficiently oxygenated (the haemoglobin will be at least 95 per cent. saturated with oxygen). In addition, the carbon dioxide carried to the lungs from the tissues will be effectively removed and vented to the atmosphere.

This process of normal ventilation can, of course, be replaced fairly effectively in patients with respiratory arrest by using a bellows like the Ambu resuscitator to ventilate the lungs with air (atmospheric air resuscitation). Provided the operator compresses the bellows often enough and with an adequate depth of stroke and maintains a clear airway, the patient will come to no harm.

It is less easy to understand how the stale expired air of the " donor " is adequate to resuscitate a patient. From Figure 104 it can be seen that expired air contains 14-18 per cent. oxygen and 4·5 per cent. carbon dioxide. This is more oxygen and less carbon dioxide than is contained in alveolar air from the depths of the lungs, since the latter is mixed with the unused atmospheric air in the air passages on expiration (dead space air). Expired air has been shown to be sufficient to maintain life in volunteers whose respiratory muscles have been temporarily paralysed with curare. The victim's arterial blood contains an adequate quantity of oxygen (the haemoglobin will be about 80 per cent. saturated with oxygen) and the carbon dioxide level remains sufficiently low over long periods of time, e.g. 40 minutes.

During expired air resuscitation the donor uses his lungs and diaphragm to inflate the victim's lungs. In this way an adequate tidal volume can be maintained.

Technique

This is best learned on one of the model patients now available, e.g. the Ambu manikin or " Resuscianne " (Fig. 105). All medical and nursing personnel should receive a course of instruction and demonstration and practise the method for themselves. The correct use of the Safar and Brook airways (Fig. 106) which facilitate the technique can be learned at the same time and also the use of the bellows resuscitator for atmospheric air resuscitation (Fig. 107).

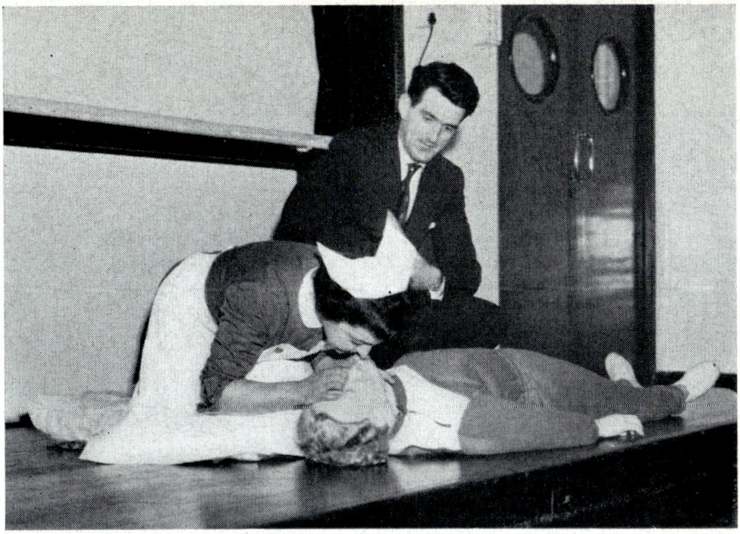

Fig. 105
A nurse practising the technique of mouth-to-mouth breathing on a manikin, under supervision.

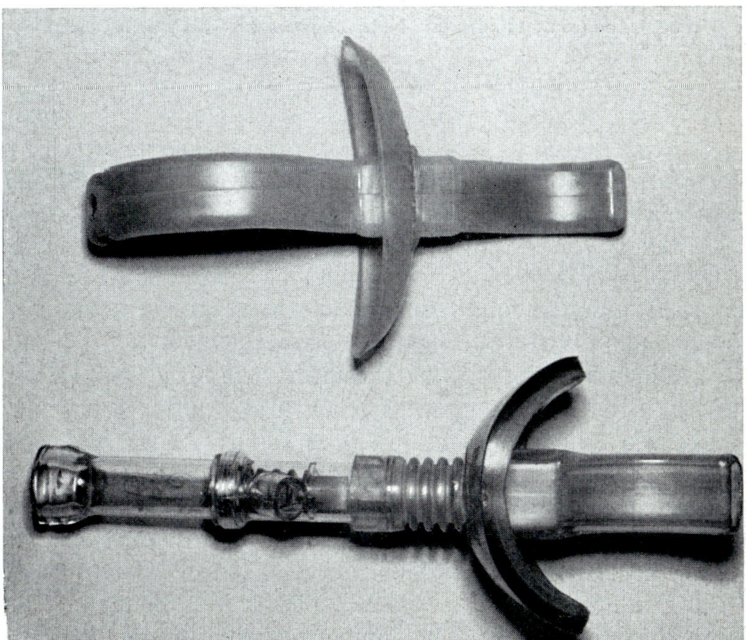

Fig. 106
Above the Safar and below the Brook airways.

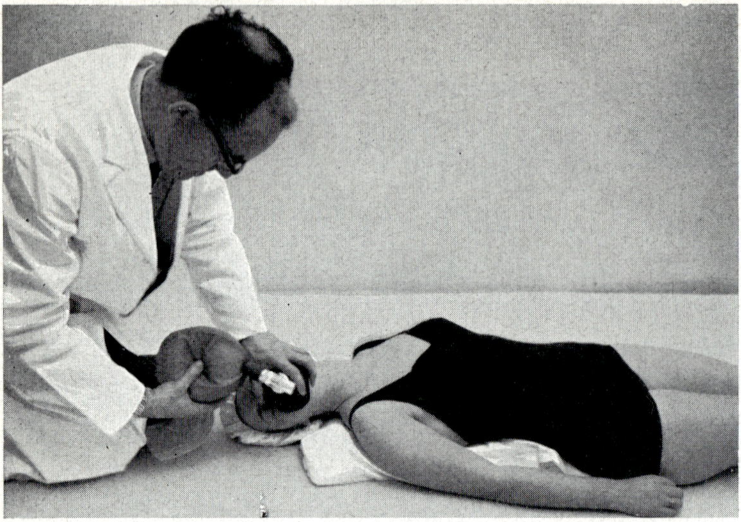

FIG. 107
The Ambu resuscitator in use. Note the position of the patient's head.

The following points must be observed:—

1. Place the victim on his back if possible.

2. Secure a clear airway by posturing the head, removing mucus from the mouth and supporting the lower jaw with the right hand to keep the tongue forward (Fig. 72).

3. Apply your mouth to the victim's, making a good seal to prevent leakage of air. In the adult, the nostrils must also be pinched with the fingers of the left hand. In the child, the donor's mouth covers the victim's nostrils and mouth.

4. Blow until you see the chest rise, removing your mouth to permit expiration. If the stomach fills with air then gentle pressure over it will empty it. The head must then be correctly postured to improve the airway and prevent a recurrence. If regurgitation of stomach contents takes place the airway must be again cleared before continuing with the resuscitation.

5. Repeat the inflation of the chest 10-20 times/minute.

6. Continue until the patient is breathing adequately for himself or further help and equipment arrive.

7. If the jaw muscles are in spasm and the mouth cannot be opened then the "mouth-to-nose" route may be employed

after the usual posturing of the head. The latter technique is, in fact, preferred by some experts in all cases.

Advantages and Disadvantages

There is only *one* apparent *disadvantage* and that is the natural reluctance of the donor to carry out a manoeuvre requiring such intimate contact with the victim. The risk of infection is minimal but in any case such a risk must be weighed against the reward of a successful resuscitation.

Advantages of Mouth-to-Mouth Breathing

The *advantages* of the method are self-evident.

1. No complicated apparatus is required.
2. The technique is easy to learn and superior to all other methods of " artificial respiration ".
3. The method is immediately available when most needed, e.g. at the scene of a drowning accident, electrocution in the home, etc.

The method is made easier if a Safar or Brook airway is available but on no account must mouth-to-mouth breathing be delayed when these airways are not immediately available. The doctor has his own " apparatus " in the form of lungs, mouth and hands.

B. EXTERNAL CARDIAC MASSAGE OR COMPRESSION

The technique is very simple and can easily be learned. Essentially it comprises intermittent compression of the heart between the mobile sternum in front and the thoracic vertebrae behind (Fig. 108). By virtue of the valvular arrangement of the heart, blood is expelled into the aorta and the pulmonary arteries following each compression (artificial systole). On releasing the sternum the heart fills with blood again (artificial diastole) from the great veins (inferior and superior venae cavae) and the pulmonary veins. The heart is compressed in a cephalad (head-wards) direction and not sideways, this latter movement being prevented by the firm attachment of the pericardium.

The following are the simple steps which make up the manoeuvre:—

1. Note the time and clear the airway. Assist ventilation if the patient is not breathing, either by the mouth-to-mouth method or with a resuscitator if one is available.

2. Place the patient on his back on a firm surface, e.g. the floor, or insert fracture boards if in bed. A soft bed prevents effective massage.

3. Place one hand palm down over the lower third of the sternum.

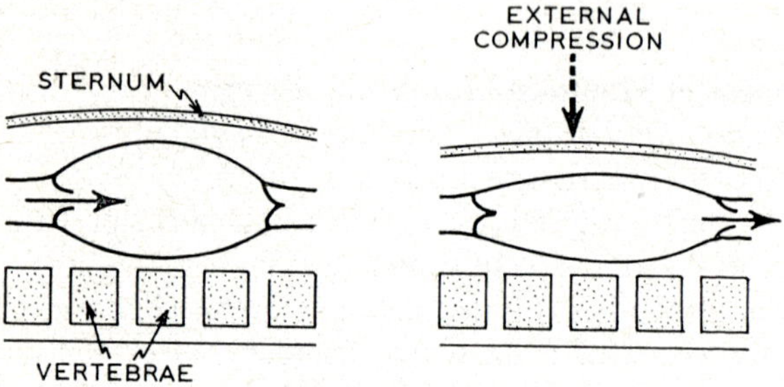

FIG. 108
This figure shows how the technique of external cardiac massage works. When pressure is applied to the sternum the blood is driven from the heart into the circulation. On release of sternal pressure the heart refills with venous blood in readiness for the next stroke.

4. The heel of the other hand is now used on top of the lower hand to compress the chest wall intermittently. The correct motion is almost a blow but with a squeezing action on the " follow-through ".

5. Repeat this sternal compression 60-80 times/minute.

6. In children it is sufficient to compress the sternum with the fingers of one hand only, to avoid undue force and damage to the chest-wall.

7. External cardiac massage is futile unless spontaneous respiration is present and adequate, or alternatively assisted ventilation is simultaneously performed.

The blood which this operation circulates *must* be oxygenated in the lungs to be of value. A ratio of 4 sternal compressions to 1 ventilation of the lungs is recommended.

On the rare occasion when the doctor or nurse is single-handed both assistance to ventilation and external cardiac massage can be performed at the one time.

During this emergency someone other than the person performing the resuscitation must send for the anaesthetist and/or surgeon in charge of the patient. They may decide to continue with the method or may institute direct cardiac massage after a thoracotomy. An ECG will determine whether the heart is arrested in asystole or ventricular fibrillation (Fig. 109). If the latter, then electrical defibrillation will be required either externally or directly on the heart itself.

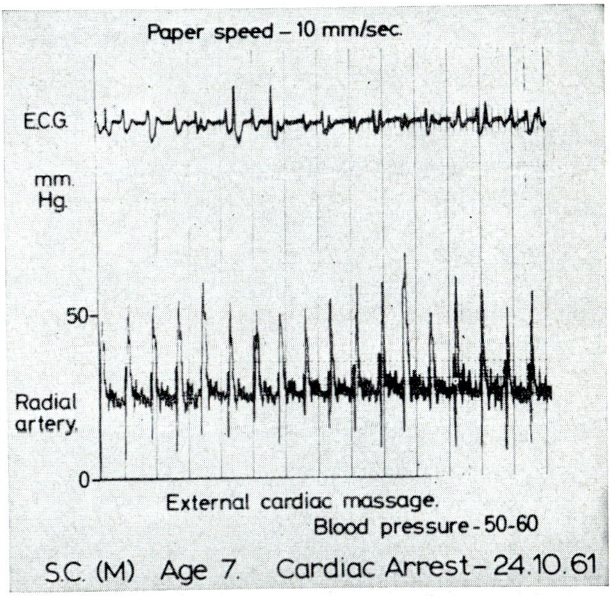

FIG. 109A

Electrocardiograms taken during cardiac massage. The upper tracings are of the ECG and the lower tracings of the blood pressure in the radial artery.
The blood pressure is maintained at 50-60 mm. Hg by external cardiac massage.

Signs of Successful Massage

1. An immediate improvement in the patient's colour.
2. Palpable carotid pulses—in time with each sternal compression.
3. Contraction of the pupils.

The resuscitation must continue until these signs of success are present and adequate spontaneous cardiac action and

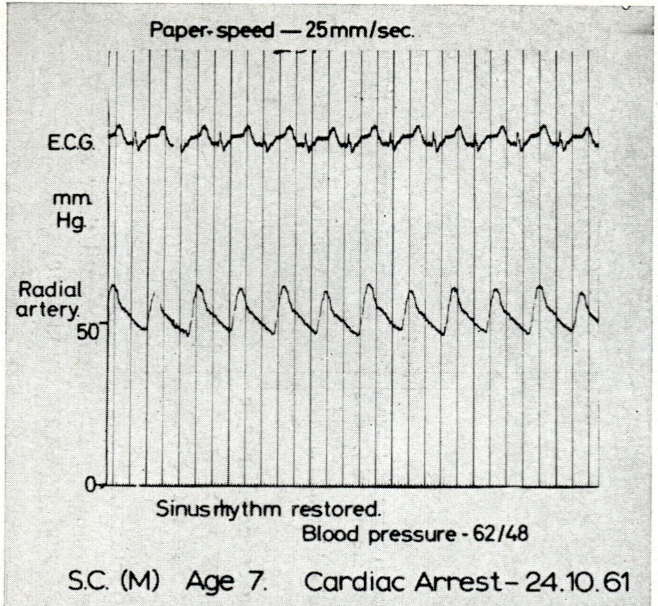

FIG. 109B

Following the cardiac massage and electrical defibrillation of the heart, normal sinus rhythm can be seen on the ECG. The blood pressure is 62/48 mm. Hg.

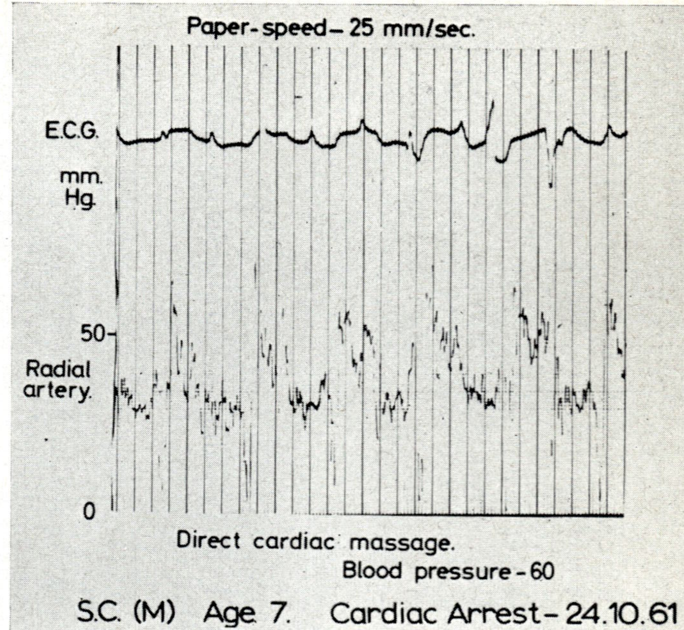

FIG. 109C

The chest has now been opened and direct cardiac massage started. The blood pressure is about 60 mm. Hg.

respiration return or until the doctor in charge indicates that hope is abandoned.

Causes of Unsuccessful Massage

There are two causes of unsuccessful massage:—

1. Inadequate Ventilation. This results in poor oxygenation of the blood returning to the heart and going to the brain.

2. Ineffective Massage. Commonly ineffective massage is caused by the subject lying on a soft surface, but occasionally it is unavoidable in thick-chested or obese individuals. Direct massage is more effective in the latter case.

To give an indication of the efficacy of this technique it should be sufficient to mention Kouwenhoven's* original series of 20 patients of all ages. Systolic blood pressures of 60-100 mm. Hg were attained during external cardiac massage and 12 of these patients are alive to date with no evidence of brain damage.

Cardiac Arrest Chart

Although there is no substitute for a thorough and continuing programme of instruction in resuscitation techniques for all medical, nursing and ancillary staff, it is generally agreed that a chart outlining the steps to be taken in an emergency is a useful aid. Such a chart includes alternative instructions for the different situations which may be encountered and guidance as to the necessary drugs and their dosage. The cardiac arrest chart should be available in all casualty departments and operating theatres and a copy should be attached to the mobile resuscitation trolley. An example of a cardiac arrest chart is included as an appendix to this chapter.

* Kouwenhoven, W. B., Jude, J. R., Knickerbocker, G. G. (1960). "Closed-chest cardiac massage". *J.A.M.A.*, **173**, 1064.

MANAGEMENT OF CARDIAC ARREST

DON'T waste time. You have only 3 minutes to establish circulation.

DON'T give drugs until type and cause of arrest is determined.

DON'T wait for E.C.G. to begin treatment. An absent B.P. and absent pulse in a major vessel means cardiac arrest.

INITIAL EMERGENCY

1. Note the time.
2. Commence external cardiac massage immediately on firm surface.
3. Commence assistance to ventilation if necessary. (Mouth-to-mouth breathing or bellows resuscitator.)
4. Send for resuscitation team and trolley. (Trolley carries E.C.G., defibrillator etc.)

DUTIES OF RESUSCITATION TEAM

(**Note:** In many cases the entire procedure can be followed without thoracotomy. Only if there is no response to the external methods is the chest opened.)

ANAESTHETIST

1. Establish a clear airway, e.g. endotracheal tube.
2. Ventilate lungs with 100% oxygen.
3. Tilt patient's head down 15 degrees.
4. Check carotid pulse when cardiac massage is established.
5. Check B.P.
6. Set up intravenous infusion as vehicle for drugs.

SURGEON

1. Continue external cardiac massage.
2. Apply external defibrillator electrodes if indicated.
3. If direct massage or internal defibrillation is indicated perform thoracotomy, i.e. open left 4th interspace transversely from sternal margin to mid-axillary line.

ASSISTANT

1. Connect E.C.G. leads to patient, confirm diagnosis, and observe E.C.G. constantly.
2. Stand-by to relieve surgeon performing massage.
3. Operate defibrillation equipment if required.

NURSES

1. Assist anaesthetist with emergency syringes and transfusion equipment.
2. Keep note of time and events.
3. Assist surgeon if thoracotomy is performed.

MANAGEMENT OF CARDIAC ARREST

POSSIBLE SITUATIONS EXISTING AFTER ADEQUATE MASSAGE AND OXYGENATION

1. THE HEART RESUMES A NORMAL BEAT

(a) Continue massage in rhythm with beat until the B.P. is maintained at a minimum of 80 mm. Hg systolic.

(b) If contractions do not improve give adrenaline 1:1,000, 0·5-1 ml. (diluted to 10 ml. with sterile water) into the cavity of the right ventricle.

(c) If contractions are fairly good but B.P. remains low give 4 mgm. noradrenaline in 500 ml. 5% glucose, slowly intravenously.

(d) In all cases give sodium bicarbonate intravenously to correct acidosis (100 m.Eq. for the average adult).

(e) If thoracotomy has been performed close chest with adequate haemostasis and water-seal drain.

2. THE HEART REMAINS IN ARREST

(A) The heart is in fibrillation

(a) Carry out electrical defibrillation external or internal and continue adequate massage between shocks.

(b) Administer sodium bicarbonate intravenously to correct acidosis (100 m.Eq. for average adult).

(c) If spontaneous beat returns follow column 1.

(d) If heart is in asystole follow column 2B.

(B) The heart is in asystole

(a) Continue adequate massage.

(b) Give calcium chloride 10%, 5-10 ml., intravenously or into the cavity of the right ventricle.

(c) Give sodium bicarbonate intravenously to correct acidosis (100 m.Eq. for average adult).

(d) If asystole persists give adrenaline 1:1,000, 0·5-1 ml. (diluted to 10 ml. with sterile water) into cavity of right ventricle.

(e) If heart beat returns follow column 1.

(f) If asystole persists continue massage up to one hour or until heart fails to fill in diastole.

CHAPTER XIII

ANAESTHESIA IN OBSTETRICS

The administration of anaesthetics in obstetric cases has many hazards, since two separate patients, the mother and the child, have to be considered. Not infrequently, the fact that an anaesthetic is required at all for some operative procedure is also an indication that neither the mother nor the child is in the best of condition for anaesthesia. Many of the indications for Caesarean section and even for forceps delivery are those involving some condition adversely affecting the foetus; for instance antepartum haemorrhage, where the placental circulation is interfered with, or prolonged labour, where there has been undue compression of the foetus, are likely causes of hypoxia in the child. In addition, the mother may be suffering from some complication of pregnancy and may have a full or semi-full stomach. The large pregnant uterus embarrasses respiration and the position on the table required for some procedures, for example forceps deliveries, is such that respiration is further embarrassed.

Before passing to the consideration of the anaesthetic techniques used in obstetric practice, it is desirable to give some attention to the problems of providing pain relief during normal labour.

Provision of Analgesia during Labour

Labour is divided into three stages, the first stage up to full dilatation of the cervix, the second stage from then until the child is delivered, the third till the placenta is delivered.

During the early stage of labour when the contractions of the uterus are felt as discomfort rather than pain, it is traditional to use mild sedatives such as chloral to control this discomfort. In some patients where anxiety is present the use of small doses of a " tranquilliser " or barbiturate may be tried. It is, however, essential to remember that when using a barbiturate in the presence of pain in such cases, excitement and restlessness may be produced.

The regular severe contractions, felt as definite and increasing pains are usually controlled by the administration of a more potent analgesic drug. The one most favoured is pethidine, given in doses of 100 mg. intramuscularly. Morphine, which is an effective analgesic and provides some degree of sedation also, has fallen from favour because of the respiratory depression which it may cause and the likelihood that this might interfere with the start of respiration of the child. It is now believed that the degree of respiratory depression produced by pethidine is almost as great as that produced by morphine, in the equivalent dosage. Pethidine is, however, claimed to facilitate dilatation of the cervix during labour and its lack of sedative properties and production of respiratory depression have been overcome in two ways.

To enhance its sedative properties it may be given with a phenothiazine drug, such as promazine, and this combination has been used with apparently favourable results by some obstetricians. To overcome the respiratory depression which it causes, pethidine has been mixed with the antagonist drug levallorphan. The value of this combination is questioned by some and, if an antagonist drug is required, it may be better to administer it separately either to the patient or to the child after delivery. Nalorphine (Lethidrone) or levallorphan may be used for this purpose. The use of uterine paracervical block for relief of pain late in the first stage of labour has much to recommend it, since depression of the foetus is avoided. This simple local analgesic technique is described in Chapter XVI.

The objections to the use of the non-volatile sedative or analgesic agents, because they produce depression of the foetus, can be minimised by restricting their use to the early part of labour, that is before the cervix is fully dilated. From then on until the child is delivered it is customary to use volatile or gaseous analgesic agents, which are rapidly excreted by the mother and should cause minimal foetal depression. The two possibilities are that nitrous oxide in air or in oxygen is inhaled or that low concentrations of trichloroethylene in air are used. In this country, midwives may administer nitrous oxide with 50 per cent. oxygen, and trichloroethylene or methoxyflurane from specially designed inhalers.

Gas and air mixtures are, however, not without hazard as the air comprises 50 per cent. of the mixture which therefore contains only 10 per cent. of oxygen. Such mixtures are therefore not suitable for patients suffering from anaemia, cardiac

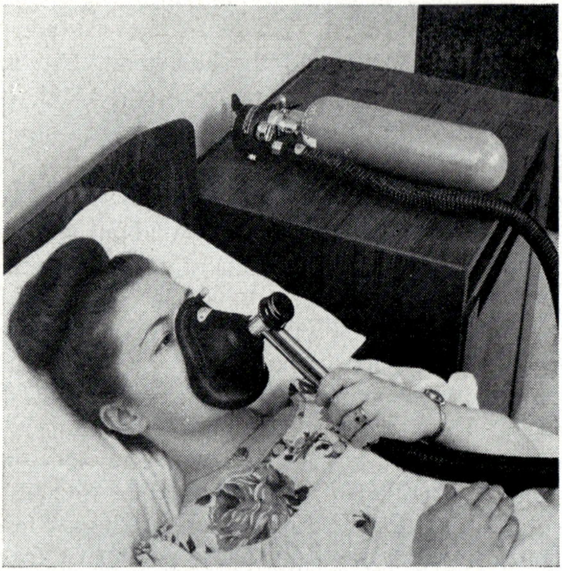

FIG. 110
The Entonox apparatus in use.

disease, respiratory disease or hypertension. The use of these gas and air mixtures is now rapidly diminishing.

The use of the more rational nitrous oxide 50 per cent.: oxygen 50 per cent. has now become much more widespread since it has been possible to combine nitrous oxide and oxygen premixed in one cylinder such that it will normally be delivered in the same proportions and supplied on demand. If the cylinder has been exposed to severe cold—and many cylinders are stored outside even in winter—the gases may separate and when the cylinder is almost empty lower proportions of oxygen are supplied. This can be prevented by inverting the cylinders several times before use. A special demand valve is used with the cylinder and the complete Entonox unit is shown in use in Figure 110.

Trichloroethylene may be administered in 0·35 or 0·5 per cent. concentrations in air from temperature compensated vaporisers which ensure that the percentage of Trilene is constant under all circumstances and this is a considerable step forward in this technique. Figure 111 illustrates the working

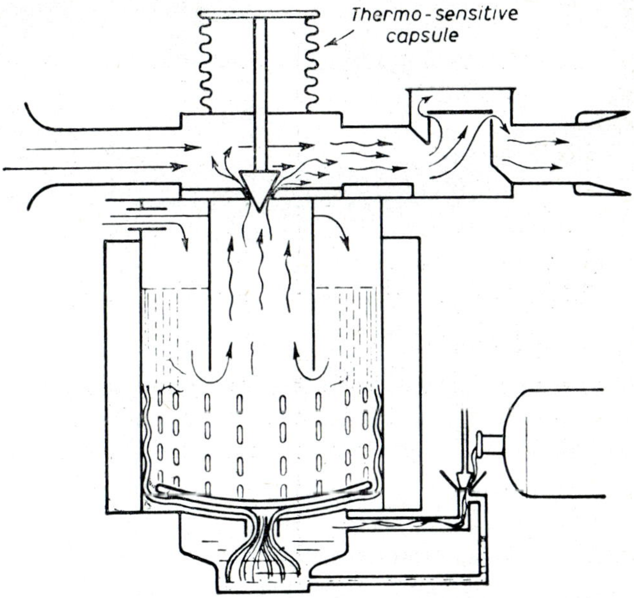

FIG. 111

Diagram illustrating the working of the Emotril inhaler.

principles of the Emotril inhaler. An inhaler working on similar lines to produce up to 0·5 per cent. methoxyflurane (Fig. 112) has been used with equally good results.

The use of these volatile or gaseous analgesics, from the stage of dilatation of the cervix to delivery of the child, is facilitated by the previous administration of the non-volatile agents which have been described. This is particularly valuable where nitrous oxide and oxygen is to be administered as the hangover resulting from opiate or pethidine supplements the weak analgesic properties of these agents. The patient should have had some antenatal instruction in the use of the analgesic apparatus and

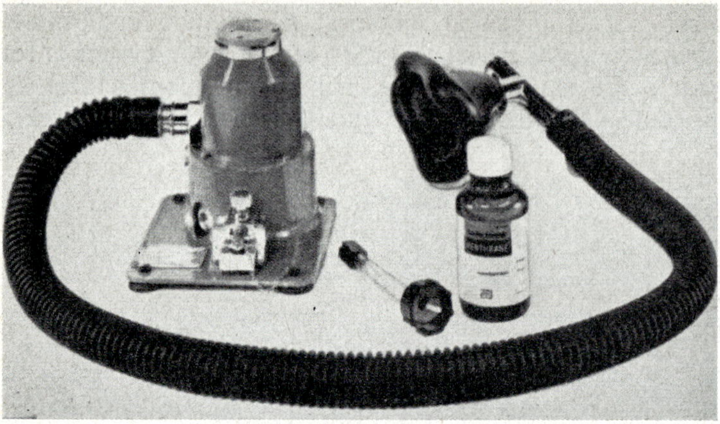

FIG. 112
The Cardiff Inhaler.

be told to take some deep breaths of the mixture with the onset of the first pain. Lack of antenatal instruction and inadequate supervision of gas and air machines have tended to discredit this technique but, where properly used, it is valuable at this stage of labour.

Hypnosis and Relaxation Exercises

The teachings of Dr. Grantly Dick Read regarding the value of relaxation during childbirth have been fairly widely accepted. Antenatal classes, where the patient is taught the technique of relaxation to be practised during the actual childbirth, are now common practice. This voluntary control and relaxation of specific muscle groups is undoubtedly of value and in many patients gives considerable relief from the pains of labour. Similarly many practitioners have found the use of hypnosis, when induced in the antenatal period and practised by the patient during labour, to be of considerable value. Hypnosis has undoubtedly some applications in this field—and some potential dangers—but when used by skilled hypnotists it undoubtedly produces good results in selected patients. It is not, however, generally considered to be an adequate substitute for other forms of analgesia.

ANAESTHETIC AND ANALGESIC TECHNIQUES IN OPERATIVE OBSTETRICS

We may summarise the problems presented by the obstetric patient as follows:—

1. The stomach is frequently full.
2. The position adopted for delivery is such that respiration is hampered.
3. In any event respiration is restricted by the presence of the pregnant uterus.
4. The depressant effect of analgesics on the foetus must be borne in mind.
5. The obstetrician, in his manipulations, may cause further embarrassment to respiration and may cause the patient to vomit or regurgitate.
6. Many patients and their babies are in poor condition when anaesthesia has to be induced.

There are many ways of overcoming these problems during operative obstetrics. The first is to employ, where possible, some form of *local analgesia.*

INFILTRATION ANALGESIA is suitable for the performance of an episiotomy or suturing the perineum after delivery. Attention must be paid to the dose employed, as the perineum at this stage is very vascular and absorption of the local analgesic from the area may be very rapid. Only dilute solutions of the chosen analgesic are required.

PUDENDAL BLOCK, described in Chapter XVI, is suitable for a low forceps delivery and may be carried out in private homes. It is a technique which should be mastered by anyone carrying out single handed obstetrics, as it is probably the safest technique for use in these circumstances, although it may be rather more uncomfortable for the patient than the use of a general anaesthetic. It is perhaps significant that pudendal block is the anaesthetic of choice in many obstetric hospitals and its more widespread use outside hospital is to be recommended.

Extradural (Epidural) Analgesia

The epidural space may be approached either via the sacral route or using the lumbar approach. Extradural analgesia is widely practised particularly in the United States and is a useful form of analgesia for obstetrics. It provides excellent pain relief and assists in dilatation of the cervix but spontaneous delivery is usually impaired and a low forceps delivery is employed. Extradural analgesia is especially valuable in cases of cervical dystocia.

Subarachnoid Block (Spinal Analgesia)

This form of analgesia has been widely used for years particularly for low forceps deliveries and for Caesarean section. It is not now a popular method of analgesia for the latter procedure. The use of subarachnoid analgesia may be associated with a fall in blood pressure which may be harmful and, if the injection spreads too far headwards, then the action of the intercostal muscles may be impaired. This is particularly dangerous where the diaphragm is splinted by the large uterus and respiratory embarrassment has been noted. This has been cited as a cause of death during the performance of caesarean section under spinal analgesia. In addition, it has been pointed out that the uterus contracts after a spinal has been given and that this may interfere with placental circulation if an unduly long time elapses between the induction of analgesia and delivery of the baby.

General Anaesthesia

In most hospitals general anaesthesia is used for operative obstetrics. The hazards associated with induction of anaesthesia in the presence of a full stomach are those which have been noted previously. Routine antacid therapy in the form of tablets given 2-hourly during labour will do much to keep the stomach contents alkaline, thus avoiding the hazards of the acid aspiration syndrome (p. 141). This is more pleasant than the single dose of 15 ml. of, for example, magnesium trisilicate which though unpalatable in a parched patient will otherwise be indicated. Where possible the stomach should be emptied before induction of anaesthesia. This may be contraindicated in cases of antepartum haemorrhage, where the retching associated with passing an oesophageal tube may cause further bleeding.

Alternatively, the patient may be postured during induction of anaesthesia.

She may either

(1) be tilted head upward and after pre-oxygenation anaesthesia induced with thiopentone and suxamethonium and an endotracheal tube passed, without previously inflating the lungs. Pressure on the cricoid by an assistant will obstruct the oesophagus and prevent regurgitation during the manoeuvre, or

(2) be placed in the left lateral position as for a forceps delivery in the classical Sims' position and anaesthesia induced and an endotracheal tube passed. Even if a tube is not to be passed, anaesthesia may still be induced in this position.

In any event the bed or the theatre table must be capable of tilting in any direction, so that either a head up or head down position can be adopted if necessary. It need hardly be stressed that, as in outpatient anaesthesia, all the normal apparatus to be found in the general operating theatre should be present in the obstetric department, namely an efficient suction apparatus, bronchoscope, anaesthetic machine and a full range of drugs and endotracheal tubes.

The choice of agents used for obstetric anaesthesia varies from centre to centre but, at present, a combination very widely used is thiopentone, suxamethonium, nitrous oxide and oxygen. Premedication is usually with atropine or hyoscine only, to avoid foetal depression. In some centres diazepam has been employed to avoid awareness during anaesthesia. After pre-oxygenation anaesthesia is induced with a small dose of thiopentone, up to 250 mg. and suxamethonium, 50 mg., is injected through the same needle. A cuffed endotracheal tube is passed and inflation of the lungs carried out with nitrous oxide and at least 33 per cent. of oxygen. The use of high minute volumes up to 14 litres/minute for 3-4 minutes will again reduce the incidence of awareness during anaesthesia as it takes time to clear nitrogen from the lungs. Intermittent injections of suxamethonium or a longer acting relaxant such as curare are given to facilitate controlled ventilation and normally no more potent analgesic is used until after delivery of the child. From then on intravenous or volatile agents may be administered. This technique is applicable to forceps deliveries, Caesarean sections and other obstetric manoeuvres, the hazards of a full stomach being present in each. Where uterine relaxation is desirable the administration of halothane for a short time may be useful.

The use of more potent volatile anaesthetic agents such as ether and halothane and the gaseous anaesthetic cyclopropane is not popular nowadays because of the effect on the foetus and on the uterus. Halothane, in particular, causes uterine relaxation and may cause considerable postpartum haemorrhage if administered in any quantity.

Despite this a light gas/oxygen/ether sequence was used for years in most obstetric units. In an emergency a practitioner familiar with this type of anaesthetic is probably safer to employ it for his obstetric patients. Most anaesthetists, however, reckon that the thiopentone, relaxant, nitrous oxide-oxygen sequence, where possible, is the better technique.

Anaesthesia for Domiciliary Obstetrics

The provision of anaesthesia for domiciliary obstetrics has always been a difficult problem. Most of the obstetric manoeuvres, however, which are carried out in a private house can be performed under pudendal nerve block. The obstetric manipulations which cannot be satisfactorily performed under this type of analgesia are probably best performed in hospital, because of the better facilities, including blood transfusions, which are available there. If a general anaesthetic must be given in a private house, there is no valid reason why the normal technique and practice cannot be carried out there, provided the anaesthetist and apparatus can be obtained. Portable suction apparatus and anaesthetic machines are available and most of the other apparatus which is required is easily transportable. Arrangements can be made to posture the patients, using pillows or an assistant if necessary and the use of the lateral position in these circumstances is recommended.

Many practitioners have for years employed simple open mask techniques, using either the ethyl chloride ether sequence or open chloroform. While these techniques, in theory, leave much to be desired and are open to potential hazards which a specialist anaesthetist would seldom contemplate, when carefully given they may suffice when no alternative is available. When using ether the fire hazard must always be borne in mind.

The other hazards of the pregnant patient are just as prominent at home as in hospital and appropriate safeguards should be employed.

CHAPTER XIV

ANAESTHESIA FOR THE OUTPATIENT

Anaesthetics for outpatients present considerable problems. Many of the patients who are subjected to these anaesthetics are unprepared and may have attended at the hospital only a short time before if at all. Often they may have a full stomach and only rarely have they had premedication. In addition, if recovery facilities are limited, the anaesthetist has to attempt to administer an anaesthetic from which there will be a rapid and complete recovery. This latter requirement is sometimes incompatible with providing ideal operating conditions for the surgeon in large, husky, patients.

Given adequate facilities for preparing the patients and a modicum of recovery beds in which the patients may lie until the full recovery of consciousness and reflex activity, the anaesthetist can do a great deal. However, even in the absence of these conditions he should endeavour to provide the same safety as he would for an inpatient in the hospital, a matter which may demand considerable ingenuity.

In cases with a *full stomach* the operation should be postponed until four hours after the patient last had anything to eat or drink. Where the operation is not an absolute emergency and the patient can be trusted, he may be asked to return to the hospital later on in the day if he has not come from a distance. Alternatively, active measures should be taken to empty the stomach by means of a stomach tube or oesophageal tube or as may be indicated. Administration of 15 ml. of an antacid may again be of value. It is important to remember, that in many of these patients, the state of the stomach may depend on the interval between the last meal and the time of accident. Thus, although a meal may have been eaten or fluid taken many hours before, if the injury has been sustained within an hour or so of the meal, the stomach may still be full a long time afterwards. This is true even in cases with injuries to the limbs with no abdominal injuries and if forgotten is a cause of trouble and sometimes even death during anaesthesia for a relatively trivial procedure. The hazards of anaesthesia in the presence of a full stomach are unrelated to the severity of the operation to be performed.

It need hardly be said that, when an anaesthetic is undertaken in the outpatient department, the normal precautions associated with the administration of an anaesthetic anywhere else should be employed. This means that suction apparatus, complete with suction catheters, a laryngoscope, endotracheal tubes and an emergency bronchoscope should be readily available. A full range of drugs, thiopentone, relaxants, inhalational agents, and the drugs normally available for cardiac arrest should be easily available.

PREMEDICATION is a problem which is normally solved by the administration only of atropine. The use of sedative premedication in the patient who is to go home is unwise, as this delays the recovery of consciousness and will make the patient unsteady on his feet after the effects of the anaesthetic itself have worn off. It is often not possible to administer the atropine one hour before the anaesthetic and it may have to be given intravenously, immediately before induction. The need for atropine is considerably reduced where non-irritant anaesthetics are used.

THE ANAESTHETIC TECHNIQUE which is employed, in cases who have a full stomach and in whom passage of an oesophageal stomach tube cannot guarantee that the stomach has been completely emptied, will depend on the skill and choice of the anaesthetist concerned. The specialist anaesthetist may preoxygenate his patient, tilt him head upwards to prevent regurgitation of stomach content and induce anaesthesia with thiopentone or propanidid and suxamethonium, apply cricoid pressure and pass a cuffed endotracheal tube. This technique is relatively safe in the hands of the skilled anaesthetist who can guarantee to introduce a cuffed endotracheal tube under most circumstances. However, for the beginner, this technique is a risky one and he is advised to select other means.

Anaesthesia may be induced by inhalational agents such as nitrous oxide, oxygen and ether. If this is done the patient retains his cough reflex and should he vomit he is less liable to inhale foreign matter. An additional safety factor may be to induce anaesthesia with the patient in the lateral position so that if vomiting does take place, the vomitus will trickle out of the mouth. This is not so difficult as it at first sounds and is a technique which is worthy of more attention.

It is worth stressing that even when a local analgesic has to be given, the danger of the full stomach cannot be ignored for, unless minute doses of local analgesic are being given, one must always bear in mind the possibility of an adverse reaction to the drug taking place, namely the occurrence of convulsions or circulatory collapse. In the former case the treatment of this condition is to administer intravenous thiopentone or a relaxant. Here the danger of vomiting and regurgitation is as great as during a general anaesthetic. However, where the stomach is full and a local analgesic can be used in small quantities this is probably a good technique to employ (Chapter XVI).

During inhalational anaesthesia in outpatients, it is possible to use a transparent mask so that vomiting and regurgitation can be seen at the earliest opportunity, and one should never under any circumstances strap the mask on to the patient's face when the state of the stomach is not known with certainty.

Rapid Recovery of Consciousness is essential in outpatient anaesthetic procedures. Often the patient is required to leave the outpatient department soon after the anaesthetic and he should do so in as co-ordinated a state as possible. Generally this means that thiopentone is not used or, if it is, only in the smallest doses. An alternative is to use methohexitone or propanidid from which the recovery is more rapid and complete than after thiopentone. Many anaesthetists, however, do not use intravenous agents at all in outpatients and prefer rather nitrous oxide, oxygen and halothane or induce anaesthesia with a 50/50 mixture of cyclopropane and oxygen as described on page 94.

The use of short acting muscle relaxants, such as suxamethonium, is popular with many anaesthetists in that fractures may be manipulated under very light anaesthesia from which recovery of consciousness is fairly rapid. Simple fractures of the forearm and leg may be dealt with in this way. However the danger of using suxamethonium in a patient with a full stomach must never be forgotten nor must the incidence of severe post-operative muscular pains. These are similar to those of influenza, with an incidence of up to perhaps 50 per cent., which discounts many of the advantages of light anaesthesia. Their incidence may be reduced where propanidid is used to induce anaesthesia although the period of apnoea following suxamethonium may be prolonged.

After the outpatient has recovered from his anaesthetic, particularly when he has had a barbiturate, care should be taken to ensure that he is sent home under supervision. In particular, he must not be allowed to drive his car home although at the time he may feel quite capable of driving. When sitting in the erect position for a period behind the wheel, he may find that he is not capable of handling a car in traffic, the medico-legal consequences of which are obvious.

In conclusion, it must be emphasised that the anaesthetic for minor operations in the outpatient must never be treated lightly, since serious complications and even death are almost as likely to follow as they are in the inpatient. As many outpatients treated for minor complaints are fit and healthy, serious anaesthetic accidents are all the more regrettable.

It has been said that minor surgery can be made perfect by treating each operation with the care that one would a major operation. The same can be said for the simplest anaesthetic; it can be made safe only by employing the full precautions one would for administering an anaesthetic for a major procedure.

CHAPTER XV

ANAESTHESIA FOR DENTAL SURGERY

In this country, more general anaesthetics are given for dental procedures than are given in all the hospitals in the country for other types of surgery.

Anaesthesia for dental surgery is the type of anaesthetic which many occasional anaesthetists are called upon to administer. It is a subject which in this book will only be dealt with in outline, as it is one which must be learned " on the job " from someone who is regularly employing the techniques to be used.

Many of the problems associated with anaesthetising dental patients are those which are found in the outpatients described in the previous chapter. However, many of the patients come by appointment and so can be guaranteed to arrive with an empty stomach. Some, a few who have been extremely nervous, may have been given mild barbiturate premedication by their dentist and this should be enquired into before starting an anaesthetic. The anaesthetist should always question the patient, before commencing the anaesthetic, regarding his general medical history and particularly if he has experienced any untoward consequences of previous dental anaesthesia. Full routine physical examination, while perhaps desirable, is seldom practicable. Premedication even with atropine is seldom employed.

Most dental patients are anaesthetised in the dental chair and the hazards of the sitting-up position have been dealt with in considerable detail by Bourne. He claims that in this position the patient may have a vasovagal attack with hypotension and faint. This hazard can be partly prevented by lowering the back of the chair so that the head and shoulders are lower than they normally would be. Ideally the operation should be carried out in the supine position.

Bourne also has campaigned for many years against the use of nitrous oxide and oxygen where anaesthesia is maintained by restriction of the percentage of oxygen in the mixture.

Nowadays *nitrous oxide* is usually administered with adequate amounts of oxygen and some volatile supplement, normally halothane. As mentioned in an earlier chapter, induction of anaesthesia with at least 20 per cent. oxygen is not significantly slower than induction with pure nitrous oxide for the first few breaths—the technique previously used.

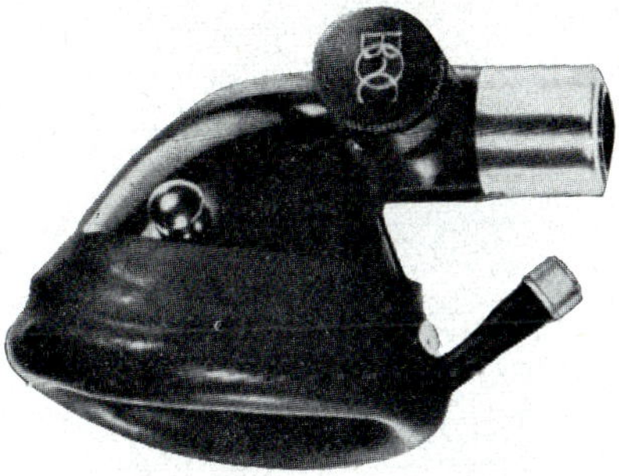

FIG. 113

A nasal inhaler such as shown in Figure 113 may be used to induce anaesthesia. A mouth gag or prop is inserted between the teeth and a pack inserted into the mouth posteriorly but not so far back as to obstruct the nasopharynx through which respiration takes place. This pack is essential not only to prevent dilution of the anaesthetic mixture by air but to prevent inhalation of blood and debris from the mouth during the anaesthetic. Concentrations of 10 per cent. and less of oxygen in nitrous oxide have been used. Such mixtures are dangerous, particularly in patients with cardiac disease, anaemia, hypertension and respiratory disease, and it is not unknown for machines set to deliver 10 per cent. oxygen to deliver considerably less while the indicator is showing 10 per cent. Bourne has drawn attention to a number of cases where recovery of consciousness has been very slow and mental impairment has followed, suggesting that cerebral hypoxia has occurred with consequent brain damage. The use of nitrous oxide and oxygen for dental anaesthesia is a technique only for the expert and many experts are abandoning this method.

Induction of anaesthesia with *cyclopropane and oxygen* has been recommended by Bourne (p. 94). Initially, he

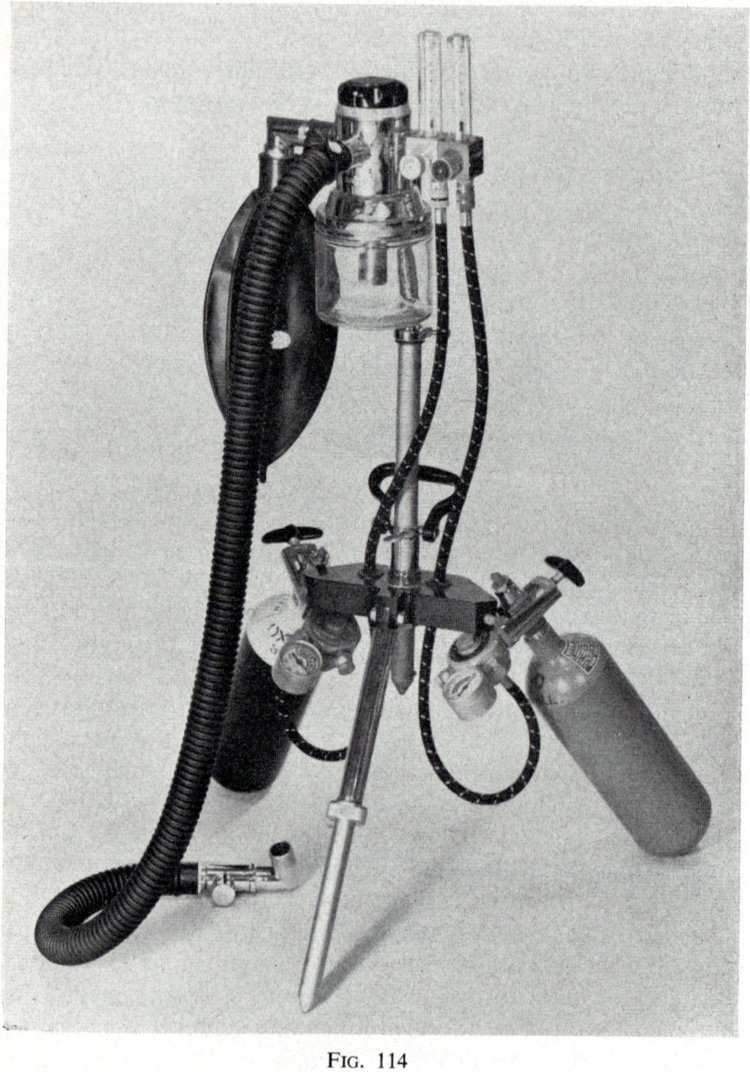

FIG. 114
The Medrex dental anaesthetic apparatus.

suggested the use of 50 per cent. cyclopropane and 50 per cent. oxygen, but it was shown that this might be inflammable when forceps were applied to teeth and the mixture now recommended has been diluted by the introduction of nitrous oxide. The reservoir bag is filled with this mixture and the patient is allowed to breathe it through a mask. When anaesthesia has been established, and this takes place in about a dozen breaths, a gag and throat pack are inserted as before and anaesthesia maintained with nitrous oxide and oxygen using 33 per cent. oxygen and halothane.

HALOTHANE as a supplement to nitrous oxide and oxygen anaesthesia has become popular in many centres and the technique described by Marrett has much to commend it. He uses the machine shown in Figure 114 and, after the administration of a few breaths of nitrous oxide and oxygen, the machine is set to deliver oxygen and halothane, the percentage of halothane being dependent on the depth of the patient's respiration. Once again when anaesthesia is established it may be maintained, if necessary, through a nasal mask using nitrous oxide, oxygen and halothane.

VINESTHENE may also be used as a supplement to nitrous oxide/oxygen.

INTRAVENOUS AGENTS: Many anaesthetists favour the induction of anaesthesia with small doses of methohexitone or propanidid. Anaesthesia is then maintained with the inhalational agents previously described. As with all outpatient procedures, adequate facilities for recovery and the return of the patient to his home must be available if other than a very small dose of methohexitone is used.

Analgesia for Conservative Dental Surgery

In some patients conservative dental procedures can be carried out more easily when the patient is unconscious or semi-conscious. To this end some anaesthetists and dentists favour techniques whereby intermittent intravenous injections of sedatives or methohexitone are given to produce a calm patient while the dental procedures are carried out. During these procedures the patients breathe air and a clear airway must be maintained while surgery is carried out. The use of diazepam intravenously as basal sedation appears to be safer than methohexitone in that laryngeal activity and the vital centres are less depressed. This technique of intravenous anaesthesia or sedation combined with local analgesia in the mouth is widespread but still controversial.

It is considered that since any general anaesthetic carries a risk, albeit small, local analgesia by infiltration or nerve block should be used where possible.

Major dental procedures should be undertaken under endotracheal anaesthesia in the same way as for any other operation on the head and neck.

Where a patient, for medical reasons, is a poor anaesthetic risk his admission to hospital where practicable should be arranged. The facilities for pre- and post-operative care and resuscitation, if necessary, will normally be better in hospital.

Finally, we would repeat that practical training in dental anaesthesia is a post-graduate study to be undertaken at the hands of experts. The Report on Dental Anaesthesia by a joint sub-committee of doctors and dentists published in 1967 by the Ministry of Health states on page 20: " We recommend that dental and medical undergraduate instruction should be based at an elementary level on the principles of anaesthesia, on the pharmacology of the drugs used and the inherent risks of their administration, on basic safety conditions and on resuscitation."

It is our hope that such knowledge may be gained from the appropriate chapters in this book and that dental anaesthesia while having special problems of its own will be based on the same principles that underlie good anaesthetic practice in other fields of work.

CHAPTER XVI

SELECTED LOCAL AND REGIONAL TECHNIQUES

The advent of the muscle relaxants caused a comparative neglect of certain well tried and useful methods of local and regional analgesia. These techniques demand a precise knowledge of anatomy and this may also explain some of their unpopularity. Recently some of these local and regional methods have enjoyed a deserved return to popularity. Before detailing the actual methods employed it would be well to consider briefly the advantages and their potential hazards.

A common misconception is that a local or regional technique is a completely safe alternative to general anaesthesia in patients who have fed immediately prior to being admitted for emergency surgery. This dangerous notion must be disposed of at the outset since there is no guarantee that the anaesthetist will not be confronted with a toxic reaction following injection of the analgesic solution.

All patients presented for anaesthesia, local, regional or general, should be fully prepared in the normal manner whereever possible. Nervous patients will usually benefit from preliminary light sedation with a suitable hypnotic. Generally speaking it is unwise to attempt these procedures in restless or drunken patients since a violent movement, when the needle is introduced to perform say a brachial plexus block, can have disastrous results, e.g. intravascular injection.

Despite the potential hazards these techniques have definite advantages to offer. They are:—

1. The minimum of equipment is required.
2. The patient can if desired remain conscious and cooperative.
3. General anaesthesia can be avoided in patients with gross respiratory or cardiovascular disease.
4. In many instances a "dry field" can be provided for the surgeon either by vasoconstriction when adrenaline is used along with the analgesic locally or, in the regional

techniques, by posturing the patient following the sympathetic blockade.

5. Prolonged post-operative epidural analgesia can be provided by continuing the analgesia with incremental doses via an indwelling catheter.

LOCAL ANALGESIC AGENTS

The drugs used as local analgesic agents vary widely in their chemical composition, some being hydroxy compounds, such as the long acting benzyl alcohol; others including procaine, are esters of aromatic acids while the remainder are a motley group including the widely used lignocaine.

The mode of action of the commonly used local analgesics is discussed in Chapter I. Being stored as water soluble salts, usually the hydrochloride, with a low pH, they react with the alkaline tissues (pH 7·4) to liberate free base thus—

$$LA : HCl + OH \rightarrow \underset{\text{(free base)}}{LA} + Cl + H_2O$$

The effect of this free base on the nerve is to stop conduction of impulses along it. This is the main effect and ideally the only one which should follow injection of these agents.

Side Effects and Toxic Effects

Some Side Effects are often noticeable after injection of local analgesic agents into the tissues or the epidural or subarachnoid spaces. It has been shown that the agent used can be detected in the blood, even in the absence of intravascular injection, and this results in a central action and the production of the unwanted effects. These are usually limited to a feeling of warmth and perhaps drowsiness due to peripheral vasodilatation and central depression. If the patient sits or stands up he may feel faint.

Toxic Effects may be manifest as restlessness, anxiety and confusion followed by twitchings, often proceeding to frank convulsions—the stage of cerebral stimulation. This may cause death by asphyxia, or may be followed by central nervous system depression with unconsciousness, respiratory depression and fall in blood pressure. These effects are due to the central action of the drug on the brain.

Sometimes, however, cardiovascular collapse may follow massive intravascular injection of the local analgesic. This is a result of direct action on the heart or blood vessels.

TREATMENT. At the stage of anxiety or slight twitching a small dose of a short acting barbiturate may be given carefully and slowly. Oxygen should also be given.

If frank convulsions have developed a short acting muscle relaxant (50 mg. suxamethonium) should be administered intravenously and controlled ventilation with oxygen commenced. The trachea should be intubated to prevent soiling with gastric contents. A barbiturate is contraindicated when convulsions have developed as circulatory depression, if not already present, would follow and be aggravated by the barbiturate.

Cardiovascular collapse of central origin or from the peripheral action of the drug is treated by vasopressors, plasma infusion and if necessary cardiac massage.

Prevention of Toxic Effects

Toxic effects are caused by:—

1. overdosage, or
2. intravascular injection, or
3. idiosyncrasy of the patient to the normal dose of the drug.

Idiosyncrasy is rare and intravascular injection can be avoided by frequent aspiration through the needle and by keeping the needle point moving during injection.

Overdosage, the most important of the three, is worthy of further consideration. There is a maximum safe dose for each local analgesic drug beyond which toxic effects will be produced. In this respect local analgesics are no different from other drugs but failure to remember this simple fact is a frequent cause of trouble. The safe dose of a local analgesic varies with:—

1. The drug used—lignocaine is twice as potent as procaine.

2. The strength of solution—the stronger solution is more rapidly absorbed and causes toxic effects more rapidly. For healthy adults (70 Kg.) we may use procaine thus.

200 ml. of 0·5 per cent.	=	1,000 mg.
75 ml. of 1·0 per cent.	=	750 mg.
25 ml. of 2·0 per cent.	=	500 mg.

3. The patient. As with other drugs reduced dosage is required in frail patients.

4. Site of injection. Absorption is rapid from vascular areas, e.g. the perineum, and it is claimed that from inflamed mucosae absorption is almost as rapid as following intravenous injection.

5. Hyaluronidase by spreading the drug increases absorption.

6. Adrenaline by delaying absorption allows a larger dose of local analgesic to be given.

A consideration of these six factors and the extent to which they apply in any individual will be valuable in establishing the maximum dose of the local analgesic agent which can be given to each patient.

The Drugs Used

There are a large number of local analgesic agents available and basically they all produce their main effect—local analgesia—and side effects as described in the preceding pages. Four agents are considered in slightly greater detail.

COCAINE, the first local analgesic used in clinical anaesthetic practice, is a vasoconstrictor unlike the other agents. It is effective by injection and surface application but is extremely toxic—four times more so than procaine. Its use is now limited to topical application for ophthalmic and ear, nose and throat procedures in a diminishing number of hospitals.

PROCAINE (Novocaine, Planocaine) was the most widely used drug in local analgesia until recently. Rapidly metabolised and only one-quarter as toxic as cocaine, it is used by injection but is not absorbed through mucous membranes except in excessive concentrations. It is therefore valueless for topical analgesia.

It has been used intravenously as an analgesic for burns dressings, to control itching and as a supplement to nitrous oxide and oxygen with a relaxant. In addition it has been used intravenously and intrapericardially to control cardiac arrhythmias during cardiac surgery.

Great care must be employed when giving procaine intravenously as toxic effects are easily produced. This is a method for the expert.

LIGNOCAINE (Xylocaine, Lidocaine, Duncaine, Xylotox). In many centres this drug has replaced procaine. It is very stable, being little affected by heat, acids, alkalis, or prolonged storage. It diffuses well, has a rapid onset of action, and a more prolonged action than procaine. It is also an excellent surface analgesic. While it was originally claimed that the maximum dose was the same as that of procaine it is now recommended that no more than 200 mg. without, and 500 mg. with adrenaline should be used in a fit 70 Kg. adult (=1,000 mg. procaine). Lignocaine 0·5 per cent. is equi-analgesic with 2 per cent. procaine and 0·25 per cent. is adequate for infiltration. Used in this way lignocaine is a safe and valuable agent.

Duration of Action and Dosage

DRUG	DOSE		DURATION OF ACTION	
	Without Adrenaline	With Adrenaline	Without Adrenaline	With Adrenaline
Procaine	500 mg.	1,000 mg.	30 mins.	1-1½ hrs.
Lignocaine	200 mg.	500 mg.	1 hr.	2 hrs.
Prilocaine	400 mg.	600 mg.	1 hr.	2 hrs.
Bupivacaine	—	150 mg.	—	5 hrs.

PRILOCAINE (Citanest) is claimed to be 40 per cent. less toxic than lignocaine, to cause less vasodilatation and to be more rapidly metabolised. However, in addition to the other side effects of local analgesics, with large doses, 600 mg. (the maximum recommended dose) to 1,200 mg., methaemoglobinaemia may occur. This can be treated if necessary by intravenous injection of methylene blue in equal dosage, but is a limiting factor to the more widespread use of this drug.

BUPIVACAINE (Marcain) is distinguished from the other local analgesic agents in common use mainly by its much greater duration of action. It would appear to be no more toxic than these other agents. In a 0·5 per cent. concentration containing 1:200,000 adrenaline this drug has proved extremely effective for " single-shot " extradural blockade in general surgical and obstetrical procedures, giving good analgesia for up to five hours.

Use of Hyaluronidase

Hyaluronidase (Hyalase) is used as a spreading agent. It is an enzyme which hydrolyses hyaluronic acid and thus speeds diffusion through the interstitial spaces. Its use speeds onset of analgesia and allows a greater area of analgesia to be produced on infiltration with a smaller volume of analgesic solution. It is of value also in plastic surgical procedures where the injected analgesic solution may distort the anatomy of the operative field.

It is not a substitute for the essential anatomical knowledge necessary for nerve blocking. Further, by increasing the rate of absorption of the analgesic it decreases its duration of action and increases the incidence of toxic reactions. It is usual to add 1,000-1,500 international units of hyaluronidase to the analgesic solution.

Use of Adrenaline

Adrenaline in dilute solution (1 : 100,000 - 1 : 200,000) is an effective vasoconstrictor when injected into the tissues. This is a valuable property when the drug is used with local analgesics as, with the exception of cocaine, they are all vasodilators. Vasoconstriction by reducing the absorption of the local analgesic agent, prolongs its action and reduces the incidence of toxic effects with a given dose. As the local analgesic drugs inhibit amine oxidase, adrenaline breakdown is also retarded.

Adrenaline is, however, a dangerous substance and must be used with great care.

Locally the vasoconstriction produced may cause ischaemic damage (see p. 264) and systemically it may cause anxiety, restlessness, tachycardia and even ventricular fibrillation and cardiac arrest. These effects can be avoided by using the drug in 1 : 200,000 concentration which is adequate and by limiting the total dose for any one procedure to the equivalent of 0·5 ml. of 1 : 1,000 solution. Stronger solutions, e.g. 1 : 80,000, are unnecessary and should be avoided. Adrenaline should never be injected round an "end artery", for example at the base of a finger or ear, the nose or penis.

PREPARATION FOR LOCAL OR REGIONAL ANALGESIA

No matter whether the method contemplated is local infiltration or subarachnoid analgesia, certain basic precautions should be considered.

Premedication

Before minor surgical procedures under local or regional analgesia, premedication is usually omitted. However, in nervous patients or for major procedures some premedication is desirable. A barbiturate is often employed to allay anxiety. These drugs in the dosage employed are ineffective in preventing the twitching and convulsions seen as toxic effects of the local analgesic drugs.

The Empty Stomach

It is desirable that even before a regional analgesic where consciousness is to be retained the stomach should be empty. Where subarachnoid or epidural techniques are to be employed, coughing and clearing the pharynx may be impaired. With less extensive procedures the risk of vomiting, or regurgitation, if toxic signs appear and have to be treated with a muscle relaxant, must be borne in mind.

Checking the Injection

The person giving the injection should check that he has the correct drug, in the correct strength of solution, and that the volume he intends to inject does not contain an overdose. He should also verify the presence or absence of adrenaline, noting the amount and strength in the volume to be injected.

Asepsis

Before embarking on an injection the administrator should scrub and, except for minor infiltrations, should don cap, mask, gown and gloves. The site of injection should be prepared and towelled as for an operation.

Explanation

It is helpful and humane to explain to the patient what you are going to do and not subject him to a series of unexpected jabs with a needle. This may cause pain, loss of confidence and a broken needle.

SELECTED LOCAL ANALGESIC TECHNIQUES

The following are some local analgesic techniques in common use. The techniques of brachial plexus block and intravenous local analgesia are suitable for use in the casualty department while pudendal block and uterine paracervical block are of great assistance to the obstetrician. Epidural analgesia has largely replaced subarachnoid or spinal block but, unlike the other techniques described, these latter are confined to specialist anaesthetic practice.

BRACHIAL PLEXUS BLOCK

The plexus is constituted by the anterior primary divisions of C5, C6, C7, C8, T1 with communicating branches from C4 and T2. These nerves first join into three trunks lying in the neck above the clavicle. Behind the clavicle each trunk divides into an anterior and posterior division and these unite in the axilla to form three cords (Fig. 115). Inferiorly the plexus is related to the first rib lying between the subclavian artery anteriorly and the scalenus medius behind. Anteriorly the scalenus anterior lies in front of the upper part of the plexus and the clavicle in front of the lower part.

TECHNIQUE. One of two techniques is commonly used—the supraclavicular approach or the axillary route.

The Supraclavicular Approach

1. The patient should be sitting or lying supine with the head rotated to the opposite side and the shoulder, on the side to be blocked, depressed. This can best be accomplished if an assistant applies gentle traction to the hand and arm.

2. Following skin preparation with a suitable antiseptic, an intradermal wheal is raised 1 cm. above the mid-point of the clavicle.

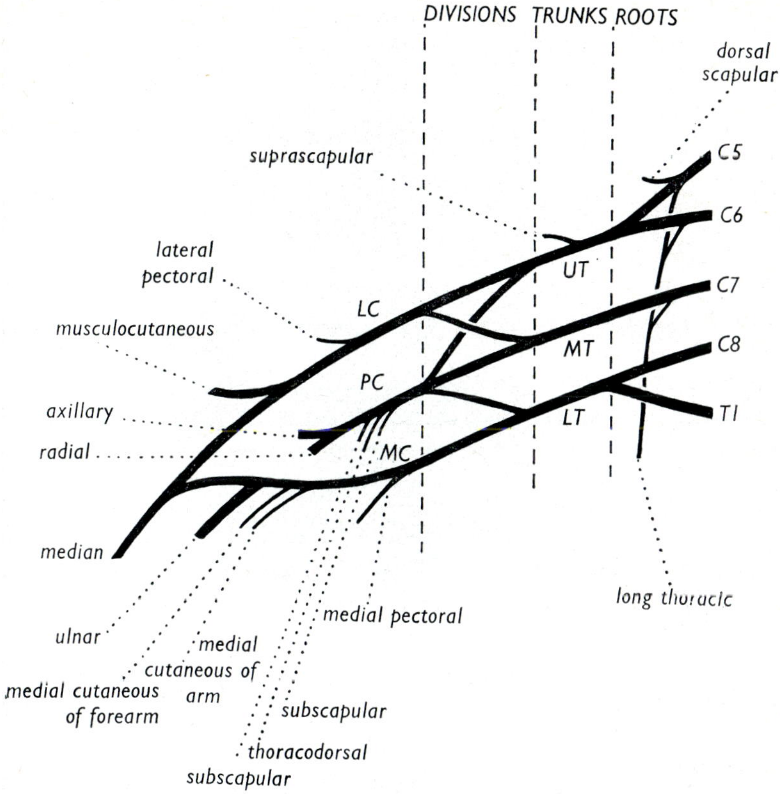

FIG. 115
Diagrammatic lay-out of the brachial plexus, U.T., M.T., L.T.: upper, middle and lower trunks; L.C., P.C., M.C.: lateral, posterior and medial cords.

3. A needle is inserted through the wheal downwards, inwards and backwards until paraesthesiae are felt by the patient.

4. If paraesthesiae are felt, 20-30 ml. of 1 per cent. lignocaine are injected following a negative aspiration test.

5. If paraesthesiae are not felt, then the needle is inserted until it contacts the upper surface of the 1st rib and 10 ml. of 1 per cent. lignocaine injected following a negative aspiration test. Three further injections of 10 ml. of analgesic solution are made between the skin and the surface of the 1st rib, each injection being 1 cm. lateral to the preceding one (Figs. 116 and 117).

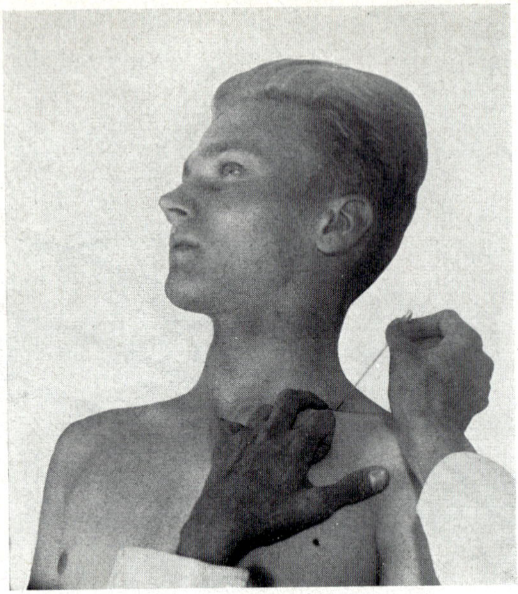

FIG. 116
The patient is in the correct position and is shown as he is seen by the anaesthetist. The patient is lying down with a pillow under his shoulders and head. The shoulder of the affected side is depressed, the head is turned to the opposite side and the muscles are relaxed.

If the patient has experienced paraesthesiae before injection the onset of the block is rapid, otherwise fifteen minutes may elapse before analgesia is complete. Motor paralysis does not always accompany analgesia, particularly with weaker solutions.

Two areas of skin are usually not analgesic, one on the tip of the shoulder and the other on the medial aspect of the upper arm. If surgery is contemplated on the upper arm, an additional ring of infiltration is required in this area.

The Axillary Approach

The main advantage of this technique is that it avoids the potential though slight risk of pneumothorax and phrenic nerve paralysis involved in the supraclavicular method. The axillary approach is also somewhat simpler.

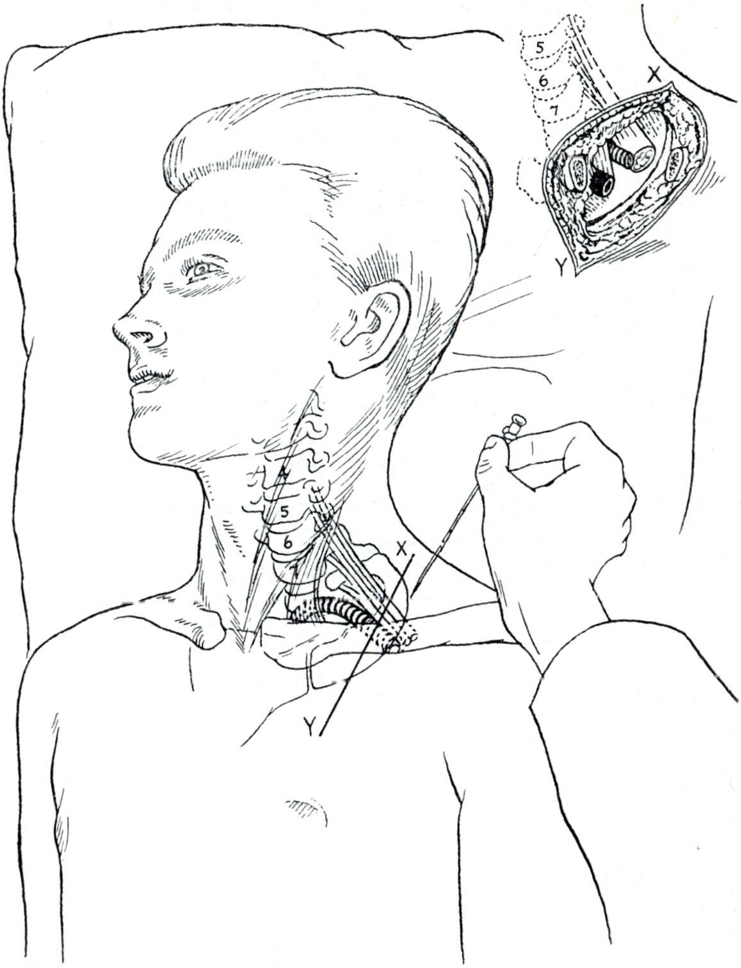

FIG. 117
The needle is directed backwards, medialwards, and downwards towards the plexus lying on the first rib. *Inset*: An incision along the line XY has been made and exposes the structures crossing the first rib. The second quarter of the clavicle has been removed.

1. The patient lies supine with the arm abducted to a right angle and the elbow flexed.

2. Following shaving of axillary hair and the usual skin preparation, the anaesthetist palpates the axillary artery as high in the axilla as possible.

3. An intradermal wheal is raised at the selected point, proximal to the lower border of the pectoralis major muscle.

4. The needle is advanced through the wheal to one side of the axillary artery, which is "guarded" by the palpating finger, until it penetrates the axillary fascial sheath. This is usually recognised as a definite click. Following a negative aspiration test 15-20 ml. of lignocaine 1 per cent., with or without adrenaline 1 : 200,000, is injected. The needle is now withdrawn to the subcutaneous area and re-inserted on the other side of the axillary artery where the injection is repeated, again following a negative aspiration test.

Just as in the supraclavicular technique, a subcutaneous ring of injections in the upper arm may be required if analgesia is desired on the medial aspect of the upper arm.

Brachial plexus block by either of these two routes, is especially suitable for surgical procedures on the forearm and hand. If a pneumatic tourniquet is used on the upper arm a "dry field" can be provided which is ideal for tendon and peripheral nerve suturing.

PUDENDAL NERVE BLOCK

The majority of low forceps deliveries can be accomplished if this analgesic technique is employed. It is particularly suited for domiciliary obstetrical practice although at present widely used also in hospitals.

ANATOMY. The pudendal nerve (S2, S3 and S4) leaves the pelvis via the greater sciatic foramen, passes across the ischial spine medial to the pudendal vessels and re-enters the pelvis via the lesser sciatic foramen. It then passes along the lateral wall of the ischio-rectal fossa in a sheath of fascia (Alcock's canal). This is the region where the nerve is most accessible for infiltration with analgesic solution.

TECHNIQUES.

1. The ischial spine is palpated vaginally with one finger.

2. The fingers of the other hand are inserted into the vagina with a 20 ml. syringe containing 1 per cent. lignocaine with 1:200,000 adrenaline held between the index and middle finger and lying in the palm of the hand.

3. The needle is inserted laterally just beyond the ischial spine to a depth of about half an inch and following a negative aspiration test for blood, 10 ml. of solution is injected.

4. The injection is repeated on the other side.

UTERINE PARACERVICAL BLOCK

This block is performed for relief of pain during the first stage of labour and is suitable for domiciliary practice. It is a simple procedure requiring only about 10 ml. of 1 per cent. lignocaine hydrochloride with adrenaline 1:200,000 infiltrated on either side of the cervix. The solution spreads in the paracervical tissues and quickly produces excellent analgesia.

SUBARACHNOID AND EPIDURAL ANALGESIA

It is convenient to consider the techniques of subarachnoid (spinal) analgesia and epidural analgesia together. In one method the drug is introduced into the cerebrospinal fluid in the subarachnoid space to produce motor, sensory and autonomic blockade by bathing the nerve roots as they leave the spinal cord. In the second method the local analgesic is introduced into the potential space immediately outside the dura mater and permeates the fatty areolar tissue there, contacting the nerves as they traverse the space (Figs. 6 and 7). The actual site of action of the drug in epidural analgesia is not precisely known but it is probable that

1. a true "spinal" is produced by diffusion of the drug into the subarachnoid space through the dura mater, or

2. the local analgesic acts directly on the nerve roots ensheathed in dura in the epidural space, or

3. the spinal nerves are blocked in the intervertebral foramina beyond their dural sheaths.

Although epidural block is technically more difficult to perform than subarachnoid block it is preferred since there is a smaller chance of grave neurological sequelae. Spinal analgesia has in the past been complicated by frequent minor sequelae such as headache and by occasional disastrous complications such as paraplegia. These unpleasant results have followed apparently uneventful and meticulous procedures carried out by experts. Although neurological complications can follow epidural analgesia these are very rare and therefore most anaesthetists prefer this technique.

Spinal Analgesia

Certain factors must be considered which influence the level of analgesia obtained when a drug is injected into the subarachnoid space.

1. THE SPECIFIC GRAVITY OF THE SOLUTION: Cerebrospinal fluid has a specific gravity of 1001-1009 at body temperature and the local analgesic is classified according to whether it has the same specific gravity as cerebrospinal fluid (i.e. isobaric), or a greater specific gravity (i.e. hyperbaric), or a lower specific gravity (i.e. hypobaric). Hyperbaric solutions will travel up or down the subarachnoid space according to whether the patient is tilted head down or head up.

2. THE POSTURE OF THE PATIENT: As mentioned above the posture of the patient during and for at least 15 minutes after injection, will influence the level of analgesia obtained. The sacral and dorsal spinal curves are sites at which the solution tends to " pool " (Fig. 118).

3. THE SITE OF INJECTION: The higher the injection site the higher will be the resulting analgesia. Generally the interspaces between L2-3 and L3-4 are chosen for hyperbaric techniques.

4. THE VOLUME OF SOLUTION INJECTED: The height of analgesia is directly proportional to the volume of fluid injected.

5. THE DOSE OF DRUG INJECTED: The higher the concentration of drug, the longer will its effect last.

6. THE FORCE AND RATE OF INJECTION: A rapid and forceful injection will result in the analgesic solution travelling further along the subarachnoid space from the site of injection.

As for most regional procedures light premedication is desirable. This allays the patient's natural anxiety and ensures a tranquil co-operative patient during the induction of analgesia. A barbiturate such as pentobarbitone (Nembutal) or quinalbarbitone (Seconal) (100-200 mg.) or an opiate such as morphine (10-15 mg.) or papaveretum (20 mg.) is convenient.

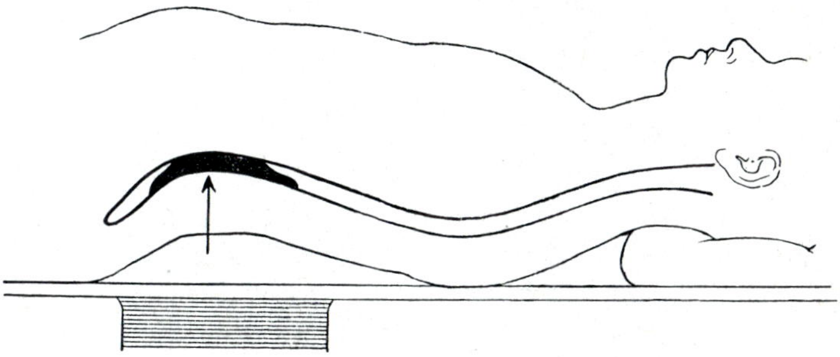

FIG. 118

When the patient rolls over on to his back the height of the lumbar convexity corresponds to the level L.2-3. The heavy solution now runs down both slopes. The part running into the sacral concavity is completely wasted as far as providing analgesia for abdominal surgery is concerned.

It is important to remember that the analgesic solution will not be fixed for about 15 minutes following injection and to avoid any movement which may result in the solution travelling too high in the subarachnoid space. The progress of the analgesia can be determined by needle-prick of the skin of the abdominal wall, keeping in mind the segmental levels (Fig. 119).

During the interval following injection the anaesthetist should set up an intravenous infusion so that a ready route for drug administration is available. If a fall in blood pressure is not desired a suitable dose of vasopressor, either intramuscularly or intravenously, should be given to the patient. Many patients are content to be drowsily awake during the subsequent surgery but their eyes should be gently blindfolded. A light general anaesthetic may be administered to others and this is usually the case with upper abdominal procedures.

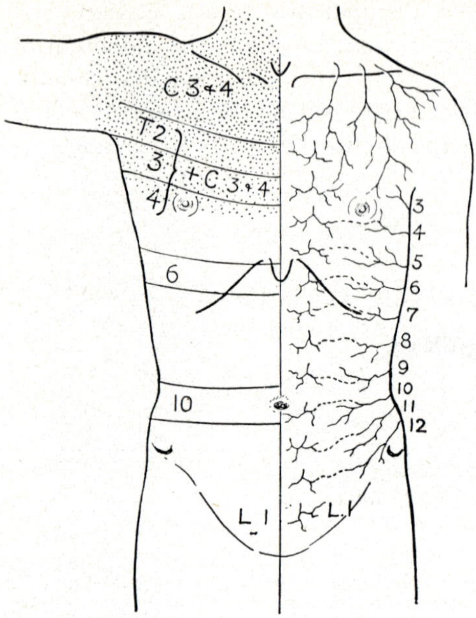

FIG. 119
Segmental levels of analgesia.

Epidural Analgesia

Subarachnoid analgesia is not popular nowadays and some of the reasons have already been mentioned. One other disadvantage is that where a high spinal block has been induced there is interference with respiration due to the muscle paralysis involving the lower intercostals. This may necessitate assisting respiration during the surgical procedure and any residual paralysis can be a danger in the early post-operative phase. Epidural analgesia, on the other hand, produces a differential block in that reflex muscle relaxation is produced without loss of motor power. This is accompanied by excellent analgesia and, if desired, autonomic block and hypotension. Although the technique is more difficult there is less chance of damage to the spinal cord. In addition, the epidural technique has many therapeutic applications outside of the operating theatre which make it a useful procedure.

The factors which influence the level of analgesia produced in an epidural block are:—

1. THE SITE OF INJECTION: The higher the injection the higher will be the analgesia. Usually the puncture is made in the lumbar region but for some purposes the upper thoracic interspaces are used. Here extreme care must be taken to avoid the spinal cord. The mid-thoracic region is dangerous and should be avoided.

2. THE RATE AND FORCE OF INJECTION: Just as in sub-arachnoid analgesia, a rapid forceful injection will result in the solution travelling further from the site of puncture and a higher level of analgesia will result.

3. THE POSTURE OF THE PATIENT: A steep head down tilt will result in the solution travelling higher and the level of analgesia will also be higher.

4. THE VOLUME OF ANALGESIC SOLUTION: Taller patients, having an epidural space of greater capacity, require a larger volume of solution if the same level of analgesia is to be obtained as in shorter patients.

5. THE AGE OF THE PATIENT: Elderly patients require a smaller volume of solution to produce any given level of analgesia.

TECHNIQUE. The patient is premedicated with barbiturate or an opiate as for spinal analgesia. The anaesthetist is gloved, gowned and masked and the patient's back is prepared as for any operative procedure. Two approaches are commonly used, one the caudal approach and the other the lumbar.

CAUDAL APPROACH. 1. The patient lies face down on the operating table or trolley with legs apart and a pillow under the pelvis. The toes should be turned inwards. This position gives the best access to the sacral hiatus.

2. The sacral hiatus, which results from the lack of fusion of the laminae of the 5th sacral vertebra and sometimes the 4th vertebra as well, is palpated. This is best done by sliding the finger upwards from the coccyx in the mid-line.

3. An intradermal wheal is raised and a straight No. 1 needle introduced at an angle of about 70° - 80° to the skin surface. This needle should not be more than 4·5 cm. long to avoid penetration of the dural sac which comes down to the level of the lower border of the 2nd sacral vertebra.

4. When the needle penetrates the sacro-coccygeal membrane, and this is usually easy to recognise, it is depressed to an angle of 15°-20° to the skin surface and it should then advance easily into the sacral canal. Two causes of failure to enter the sacral canal are:—

(*a*) The needle may be advanced superficial to the hiatus and the injection made subcutaneously with resulting swelling at the site of injection.

(*b*) The needle may be inserted under the periosteum.

5. Following a negative aspiration test for cerebrospinal fluid and blood, a test dose of 5 ml. of 1·5 per cent. lignocaine without adrenaline is injected.

6. If no motor paralysis is evident after a period of five minutes, when the patient has been asked to move his toes, the rest of the injection is proceeded with. About 20 ml. of 1·5 per cent. lignocaine is required for anal fissure operations or haemorrhoidectomy. The analgesia is complete in ten minutes and lasts about one hour.

The anatomy of the caudal space is variable and the space may be loculated. This can result in unilateral analgesia.

LUMBAR APPROACH. To reach higher levels from the caudal approach larger volumes of analgesic would be required with a greater risk of toxic effects. The lumbar approach is therefore preferred for abdominal procedures. A special needle, the Tuohy needle, is used for a lumbar epidural analgesia (Fig. 120).

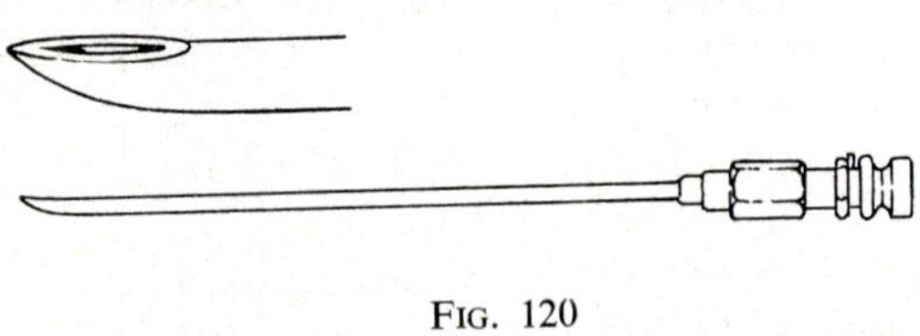

FIG. 120

The Tuohy needle. The trocar point and side opening can be seen.

A catheter introduced through the Tuohy needle, directed up or downwards by rotation of the needle, enables a continuous epidural analgesia to be administered. The catheter can be connected to a paediatric " burette type " intravenous set thus ensuring absolute sterility.

This modification enables post-operative analgesia to be continued for hours or in some cases days and is a useful method in patients with severe respiratory disorders. The same technique, or the continuous caudal alternative, can be employed in labour particularly in cases of cervical dystocia. Other therapeutic indications for continuous epidural analgesia are for the relief of pain in acute pancreatitis, for the relief of pain and autonomic blockade in peripheral vascular disease and arterial embolism in the legs.

Control of Blood Pressure

The autonomic blockade which follows epidural analgesia results in hypotension. This can be of great advantage to the surgeon, providing a fairly bloodless field for major procedures such as Wertheim's hysterectomy, but it must be controlled. The blood pressure must not be permitted to fall below 60 mm. Hg. in fit patients and any blood loss must be meticulously restored. Should hypotension be contra-indicated, a vasopressor such as methoxamine (5-15 mg.) can be given intramuscularly following completion of the epidural injection.

INTRAVENOUS REGIONAL ANALGESIA

This technique is at present enjoying a revival, and deservedly so, because of its simplicity and safety. First described by Bier in 1908 it is a useful method of analgesia for emergency surgery on the limbs. For operations on the arm and hand it is preferred by many to brachial plexus block which requires a greater degree of technical skill to accomplish and has occasional complications such as pneumothorax.

METHOD. A standard sphygmomanometer cuff, or a specially designed double cuff (Fig. 121), is placed round the patient's arm and the systolic blood pressure recorded. A needle or disposable plastic cannula is then introduced into a vein on the back of the hand, or forearm if the hand is involved in the injury. The limb is raised and emptied of blood by the application of an Esmarch bandage, applied from the hand proximally to the level of the blood pressure cuff which is then inflated to just above the systolic pressure. Forty ml. (in a healthy 70 kg. adult) of 0·5 per cent. lignocaine without adrenaline is then injected into the needle or cannula for an arm (i.e. 200 mg. lignocaine) or up to 100 ml. for a leg (i.e. 500 mg. of lignocaine). Paraesthesiae usually develop during the injection and are immediately followed by profound analgesia and frequently complete muscle paralysis.

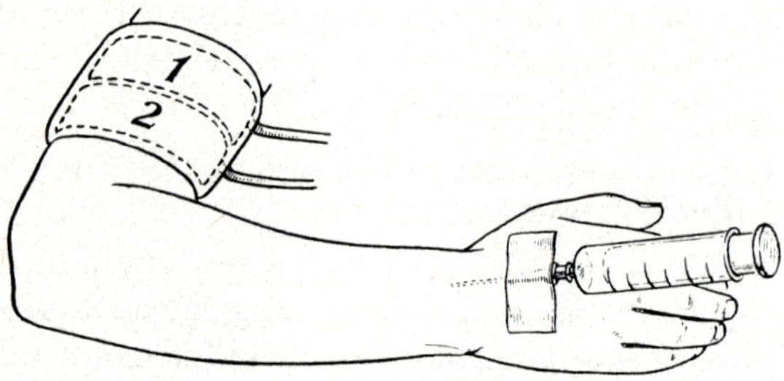

FIG. 121
Intravenous local analgesia. The upper cuff is inflated after the limb has been rendered bloodless. The injection is then made, the lower cuff inflated and finally the upper one deflated.

On completion of the surgical procedure power and sensation return to the limb within five to ten minutes of release of the tourniquet.

ADVANTAGES

1. A suitable technique for emergency procedures in patients not prepared for general anaesthesia.
2. The technique is extremely simple and reliable.
3. The risk of complications is much less than with brachial plexus block.

CHAPTER XVII

TECHNIQUES ASSOCIATED WITH ANAESTHESIA

HYPOTHERMIA IN ANAESTHESIA

Moderate hypothermia, i.e. 28 to 32° C., is used clinically in two ways. It may be used in the *treatment of hyperpyrexia* when the body temperature increases to dangerous levels. This situation is met with following some head injuries and also following allergic reactions to drug therapy. The second clinical use of body cooling is in cardiovascular surgery, where certain operations can be performed during *temporary occlusion of the circulation.* The hypothermia protects the brain and other organs, for a limited period of time, from the effects of hypoxia. This is possible since the basal oxygen requirements of these tissues are reduced at low temperatures (Fig. 122).

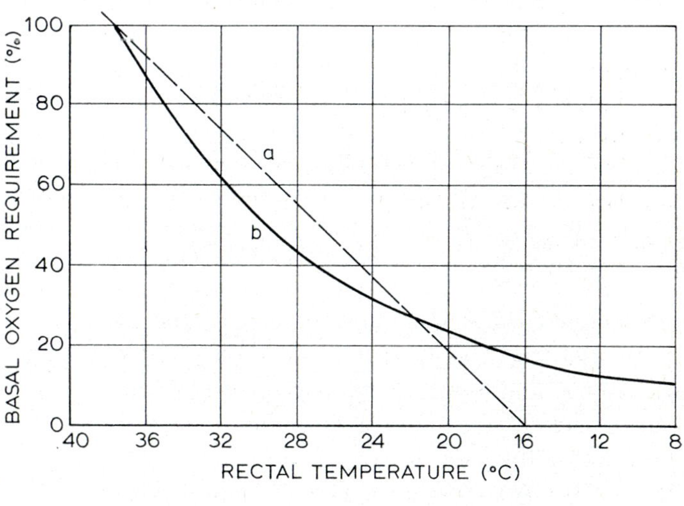

FIG. 122

The fall in oxygen requirement of the body with fall in temperature was thought to be a linear relationship (a), but is now known to be exponential (b).

Since the anaesthetist may require to induce hypothermia in the intensive care unit during the management of head injuries, as well as in the cardiovascular theatre, some of the methods available are mentioned here.

Methods

Outside the operating theatre the technique of body surface cooling is the one commonly employed and this can be accomplished in many different ways. The following are some of the methods in use.

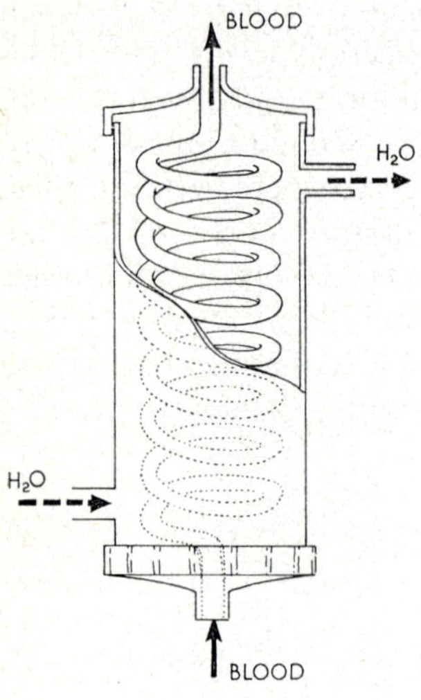

FIG. 123

A heat exchanger. The circulating blood passes through the coil and is cooled or heated by water in the surrounding jacket.

1. ICE-BAGS: The application of ice-bags to the patient's skin surface in the axillae, around the neck and in the groins is the simplest technique available. These sites are chosen because major arteries lie close to the surface and the blood is more readily cooled.

2. IMMERSION COOLING: The patient can be immersed in a bath of water at a temperature of 15 to 18 °C. The water is circulated over the body surface and this is a very effective cooling technique.

3. COOLING BLANKET: Special blankets containing a "cooling coil" can be wrapped around the patient. A coolant like ethylene glycol or cold water is circulated through the coil.

4. WATER SPRAY COOLING: Cold water is sprayed on to the skin surface and returned to a reservoir, from which it is pumped back to the spray again. This is really a variant of immersion cooling and equally effective.

5. SURFACE AIR COOLING: This technique requires a cooling cabinet through which cold air is blown by a fan and circulated over the patient's skin. This method permits of greater precision in attaining the desired degree of cooling.

Although any of the techniques described above can be used prior to cardiac surgery, the method generally preferred nowadays is blood-stream cooling. Here the patient is connected to a heart-lung machine combined with a heat-exchanger which cools or warms the circulating blood as it is delivered to the patient from the oxygenator (Fig. 123).

Temperature Measurement

The phrase " body temperature " lacks precision and it is important to state the site at which any temperature reading is taken, e.g. oral, rectal, oesophageal or nasopharyngeal. During induced hypothermia, temperature gradients are set up throughout the body, since cooling of the tissues is not uniform. The body " core " is warmer than the skin surface and the brain may be at a different temperature from the liver.

In order to control the cooling process properly, continuously recording thermometers capable of reading to low levels should be employed and not the usual mercury glass clinical type. Figures 78 and 79 show two types of thermometer which are suitable.

Control of the Cooling Process

The normal body reaction when exposed to cold is vasoconstriction and shivering. This protective mechanism must be overcome if hypothermia is to be controlled. This is done by employing drugs which act centrally on the thermal nucleus in the hypothalamus and on the shivering centre in the thalamus. General anaesthetic agents and the phenothiazine drugs act in this way and assist the cooling process. Peripherally acting drugs, which prevent the muscle fibrillation and vasoconstriction found during shivering, may also be employed. The general anaesthetic agents again act in this way as do the curariform and ganglion blocking drugs.

When the active surface cooling process is stopped, the core temperature of the body continues to fall due to redistribution of heat in the body (Fig. 124). This " after-drop " in temperature must be anticipated by stopping the cooling process in good time, otherwise the core temperature may fall below 28 °C. Below this level cardiac arrhythmias are common and spontaneous ventricular fibrillation can occur (Fig. 125). If ventilation is not controlled, when the body temperature falls to the region of moderate hypothermia, respiration becomes inadequate and the arterial carbon dioxide content rises with a resultant fall in pH. This respiratory acidosis occurs despite the reduction in carbon dioxide production that accompanies tissue cooling

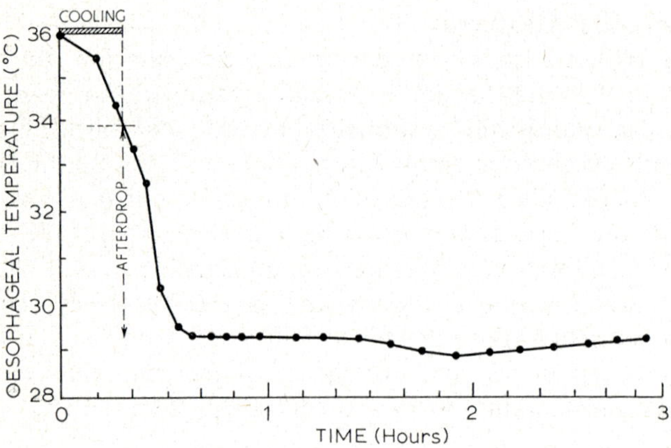

FIG. 124
A cooling chart showing the fall in temperature after active cooling has stopped—the after-drop.

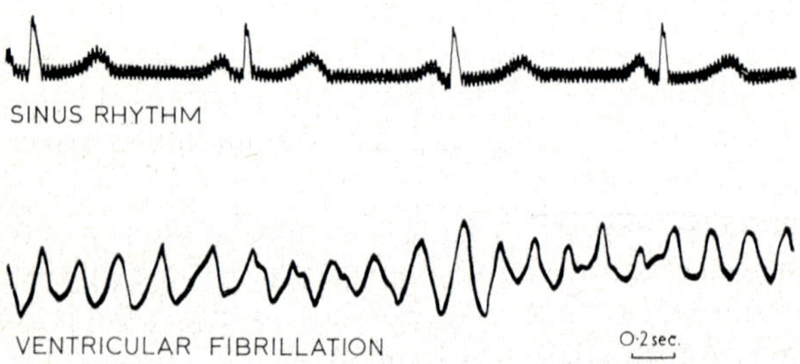

FIG. 125
Electrocardiograms of sinus rhythm and ventricular fibrillation.

If hypothermia is to be a controlled process, it is evident that careful attention must be paid to the cardiovascular and respiratory state as well as to continual recording of the temperature at various sites in the body.

INDUCED HYPOTENSION IN ANAESTHESIA

For many surgical procedures a bloodless field is a great advantage. This is particularly true of plastic surgery and neurosurgery, but, since there are definite risks associated with the technique, generalised hypotension should not be employed unless it is essential to the success of the surgical procedure. It should never be undertaken lightly but only after careful consideration of the patient's fitness for the procedure. Hypotension carries an increased risk where there is evidence of coronary or cerebral ischaemia or where hepatic or renal function is abnormal.

Methods

1. Total Spinal Analgesia: Sympathetic blockade with resulting hypotension can be produced by the subarachnoid injection of a local analgesic agent such as cinchocaine or lignocaine.

2. High Epidural Analgesia: Sympathetic blockade is produced by the injection of local analgesic solution in the epidural space.

3. Ganglion Blocking Drugs: Sympathetic blockade can be produced by the intravenous administration of drugs such as hexamethonium (Vegolysen) or trimetaphan (Arfonad). This is also obtained when curare and halothane are administered together.

4. Controlled Arteriotomy: This technique is little used nowadays. The blood pressure is lowered by reduction of the circulating blood volume, the blood being replaced by transfusion at the end of the operation.

Anaesthetic Technique

Whatever method is used to induce hypotension, the accompanying anaesthetic technique must be meticulous. Adequate oxygenation must be ensured throughout the procedure and respiration supported if at all inadequate. Although bleeding is reduced during surgery, accurate assessment of any blood loss and immediate replacement is essential, if normal blood pressure is to be successfully restored after the operation.

Hypotension can only be considered as " controlled " if close attention is paid to the aforementioned points and if the blood pressure is constantly and accurately measured. The systolic blood pressure should not be permitted to fall below 60-70 mm. Hg or renal damage with resulting post-operative renal failure may occur. The blood pressure can be adjusted by altering the patient's posture, e.g. raising the lower limbs or by giving a vasopressor drug such as methoxamine.

Post-operatively the patient must be nursed supine until the effects of the sympathetic blockade wear off. Blood pressure readings should be made frequently, for the first hour or two post-operatively, until stable readings are obtained at the pre-operative values.

NEUROLEPTANALGESIA

Certain minor neurosurgical procedures and diagnostic procedures, such as cardiac catheterisation, may ideally be performed in patients who are sedated and free from pain, where muscular relaxation is not essential. The patient's co-operation is occasionally required during the procedure and therefore he or she should be capable of being aroused. This state of sedation and indifference to environment, combined with analgesia and the ability to co-operate when required, is known as neuroleptanalgesia. As yet, no one drug can produce these conditions, but various combinations have been tried with more or less success.

The technique is based on the combination of a neuroleptic drug, producing sedation or indifference to the environment, with a potent analgesic. The potent analgesics used, phenoperidine and fentanyl are pethidine like drugs and in large doses have similar disadvantages, namely respiratory depression, nausea and vomiting. The first of the neuroleptic drugs used, haloperidol, produced a fairly high incidence of side effects in the form of hallucinations and extra-pyramidal reactions. More recently dehydrobenzperidol (Droperidol) has been used but in larger doses it may also cause these unpleasant side effects. Evidence has also been produced to show that while some of the patients lie apparently calm and sedated they are experiencing hallucinations.

These side effects have so far limited the use of the technique. In this field research is continuing and there is no doubt that exciting developments may be expected in the future.

ELECTRONARCOSIS

The question, " Why is a drug an anaesthetic and how does it work?" is often asked. There is no doubt that the final answer is not yet available, since many diverse drugs can produce anaesthesia although apparently acting in quite different ways. In addition, various physical means of producing insensibility and freedom from pain are known and, for many years, it has been apparent that electrical currents passed through the brain can produce unconsciousness and freedom from pain for short intervals, e.g. during electroconvulsive therapy. This approach has enjoyed a revival recently and anaesthesia or electronarcosis produced in this way is being used in some centres.

The advantages of this technique are obvious in that, since no drug is administered, there is no concern about liver function and renal function with regard to drug elimination. Respiratory and cardiovascular depression are minimal and post-operative recovery is rapid and free from drug " hangover ". Although the method is not yet widely accepted, it is attractive enough to warrant further trial and investigation.

CHAPTER XVIII

THE ANAESTHETIST IN CONSULTATION

By virtue of his special knowledge of the management of respiratory problems in the operating theatre and his familiarity with a wide range of drugs and their antidotes, the anaesthetist has a role to play outside the traditional confines of the operating theatre. His advice and technical assistance may be required in the management of therapeutic problems which fall broadly into two groups.

The first group is where *intractable pain* is a problem, e.g. in terminal carcinoma: tic douloureux etc. Here he can often help, because of his familiarity with the techniques of local analgesia. The injection of solutions of local analgesic into the epidural or subarachnoid spaces can also be used to relieve severe pain and, in terminal carcinoma of the pelvic organs, a *permanent block* can be performed by injecting a solution of *phenol* or *alcohol* into the extra-dural space, destroying all pain-carrying fibres from the affected area. In some hospitals " pain clinics " have been established under the general supervision of the anaesthetic department.

The second group of problems with which the anaesthetist has to deal are *respiratory in origin*. The anaesthetist is using techniques involving the control of respiration daily and is constantly measuring and assessing respiratory function. These respiratory problems may arise pre-operatively or post-operatively or may be unassociated with any surgical problem, e.g. poliomyelitis or severe myasthenia gravis.

The common causes of surgical respiratory problems fall readily into five groups.

1. Pre-existing Lung Disease

Pre-existing lung disease, unrecognised pre-operatively is one of the commonest causes of post-operative respiratory failure. Patients with chronic obstructive lung disease usually suffer from acute exacerbation of their disease during the winter months and are always on the verge of lung failure.

Even minor surgery, requiring general anaesthesia, can have a similar effect and result in acute respiratory failure. It is very important that such patients should, whenever possible, have pulmonary function tests and blood gas analyses performed pre-operatively in order to assess the severity of their disease and thus the advisability of surgery. If operation is essential, the particular anaesthetic technique best suited to them can be chosen. When elective surgery is contemplated there is time for full investigation and to institute a prophylactic régime of antibiotics, broncho-dilator drugs, postural drainage and physiotherapy. A " prophylactic " tracheostomy may be indicated. General anaesthesia may be contra-indicated and many procedures can be done under epidural or regional analgesia instead.

There are two other types of patient who may be conveniently discussed here. The first is the grossly obese patient with respiratory embarrassment. Here the lungs themselves may be normal but the patient suffers from dyspnoea on exertion, due to the increased oxygen demands resulting from the effort of maintaining mobility. Further disablement results from poor muscle tone in the respiratory musculature and " splinting " of the diaphragm by the abdominal contents. These patients must be dieted rigorously pre-operatively and physiotherapy can be of assistance.

The second type of case is the patient suffering from constrictive disease of the thorax, e.g. ankylosing spondylitis, where again the lungs may be normal but the respiratory excursion of the thorax severely limited. Regional or epidural analgesia is again preferred here for intra-abdominal surgery.

The quick return of an active cough reflex post-operatively is particularly important in all patients with pre-existing lung disease, in order that secretions may not accumulate in the bronchi giving rise to the typical " post-operative chest ", i.e. atelectasis or pulmonary collapse and pneumonia (Fig. 126).

2. Traumatic Conditions

Patients with multiple injuries may first present as acute respiratory problems. For instance, a severe facio-maxillary injury often has upper airway obstruction and is in imminent danger of asphyxiating unless a clear airway is secured before

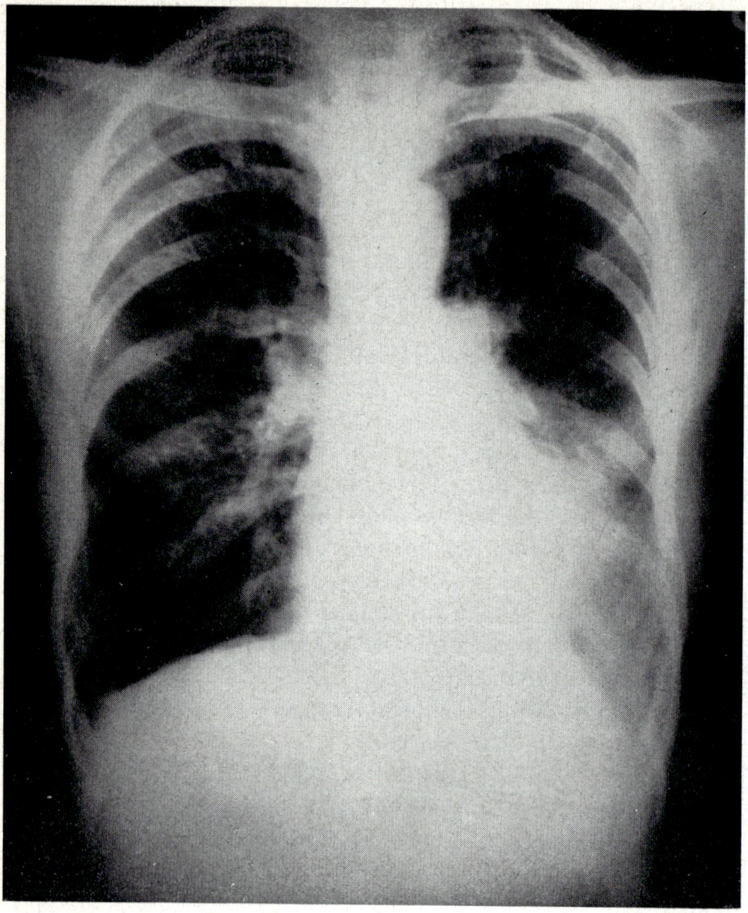

FIG. 126
A radiogram showing atelectasis of the lower lobe of the left lung.

surgery is contemplated. In an emergency, an endotracheal tube may be introduced and oxygen, with perhaps assistance to ventilation given. A tracheostomy may then be performed if there is doubt about maintenance of the airway, after corrective surgery is completed (Fig. 127).

Patients with severe head injuries, in deep coma, are in grave danger of obstruction of the airway either from the tongue falling back against the posterior pharyngeal wall or by inhalation of regurgitated gastric contents while the cough reflex is depressed. At an early stage the airway should be secured by means of an endotracheal tube or tracheostomy and the stomach emptied. Damage to the vital centres, including the respiratory centre, may cause inadequate respiration or occasionally apnoea may ensue. This is an indication for assistance to ventilation either by hand or by a mechanical ventilator.

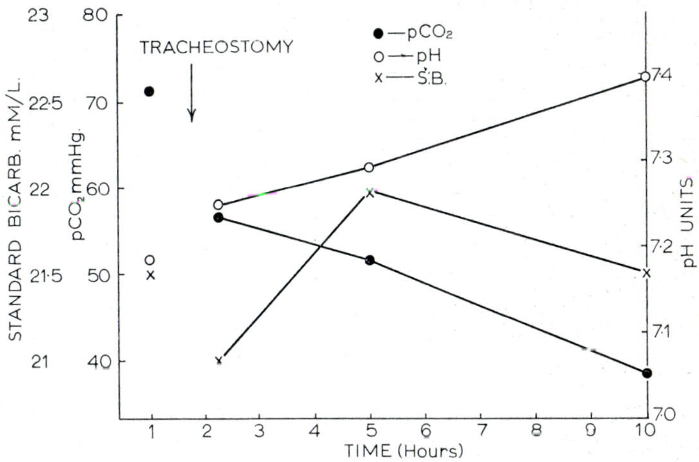

FIG. 127

The effect on the arterial blood gases of a tracheostomy in a patient with respiratory acidosis. The arterial carbon dioxide tension level fell with the improvement in alveolar ventilation and the pH rose to normal.

Trauma to the chest wall—the " crushed chest " or " stove-in-chest "—is worthy of special mention. This high velocity impact injury is becoming increasingly common in car accidents. As a result of this injury a segment of the thoracic wall, most frequently lateral but occasionally anterior, is floating free due to rib fractures anteriorly and posteriorly (Fig. 128). The underlying lung is also contused and there may be a pneumothorax or haemopneumothorax. In the worst examples of this the patient presents in acute respiratory failure with grave hypoxia and hypercarbia.

What happens when such a patient tries to breathe spontaneously?

(*a*) On inspiration the thoracic cage expands but the floating segment is sucked in. On expiration the thorax retracts and the floating segment is pushed out.

(*b*) An additional effect is that of mediastinal shift leading to a reduction in central venous return and consequent reduction in cardiac output and heart failure.

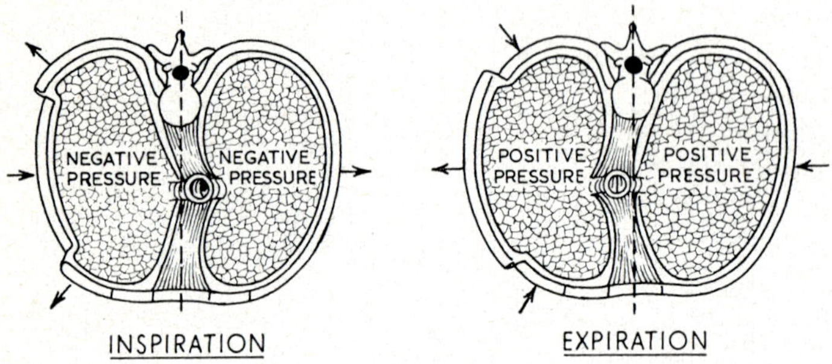

FIG. 128

The "crushed-chest" injury. The paradoxical movement of the damaged chest wall and the movement of the mediastinum during respiration can be seen.

(*c*) Interpulmonary "shunting" of gas occurs so that, on inspiration, the fresh gas entering the intact lung is diluted with gas low in oxygen but high in carbon dioxide from the damaged side. On expiration some of the gases from the intact lung enter the damaged side instead of being vented to atmosphere.

(*d*) The alveoli in the damaged lung are unable to take part in normal ventilation resulting in hypoxia and hypercarbia. This latter factor is probably the most important single cause of respiratory failure in these patients.

It is obvious that this state of acute respiratory failure must be treated quickly and adequately before any surgery is embarked upon. Immediate endotracheal intubation with I.P.P.V. and oxygen and insertion of a water-sealed drain on the damaged side (in case of tension pneumothorax and to drain the haemothorax) is essential. Later a tracheostomy may be performed as many of these patients require prolonged mechanical assistance to ventilation. I.P.P.V. with oxygen reverses most of the ill-effects of the crushed chest immediately, e.g. paradoxical respiration and shunting of gas in the lungs, and an immediate clinical improvement is usually obvious. In very few of these cases of crushed chest injury is surgery indicated, such as wiring ribs or applying external traction. In most cases I.P.P.V. and the measures described are sufficient by themselves.

3. Surgery on Lungs and Airway, etc.

It is obvious that, in a patient already suffering from lung disease, removal of diseased lung, with inevitably some normal lung tissue as well, as in lobectomy and pneumonectomy, may result in respiratory failure. The effect of removal of one or other lung in such a patient can often be predicted pre-operatively by differential bronchospirometry. Here lung function studies can be carried out on each lung separately and the result of removal of one or other lung predicted.

Surgery in the neck, e.g. thyroidectomy, can present some problems so far as respiratory function is concerned. In malignant disease of the thyroid or in thyroiditis, e.g. Hashimoto's disease, the gland may obstruct the underlying airway. This results in narrowing of the airway—" scabbard trachea " —and there may be a marked respiratory stridor. Tracheostomy under local analgesia before the thyroidectomy, is occasionally necessary and cases occur where a tracheostomy is required post-operatively, due to complete respiratory obstruction resulting from damage to the recurrent laryngeal nerves.

4. Abnormal Response to Drugs and Drug Overdose

An interesting group of patients who come to surgery are those suffering from a variety of relatively rare conditions which may have been diagnosed before surgery for some other coincident disease, e.g. myasthenia gravis, porphyria and a genetically transmitted condition in which a plasma enzyme, pseudocholinesterase, is deficient.

Patients with myasthenia gravis are abnormally sensitive to the competitive or non-depolarising muscle relaxants commonly used during anaesthesia. A prolonged post-operative respiratory muscle paralysis results requiring mechanical assistance to ventilation until the drug effect wears off.

In porphyric patients, the use of barbiturates for induction of anaesthesia can result in an acute exacerbation of the condition with respiratory muscle paralysis post-operatively and again prolonged mechanical assistance to ventilation will be required.

Another relaxant drug commonly used during anaesthesia is suxamethonium which normally has a short action, being destroyed by an enzyme called pseudocholinesterase occurring in normal plasma. One group of patients have either an ab-

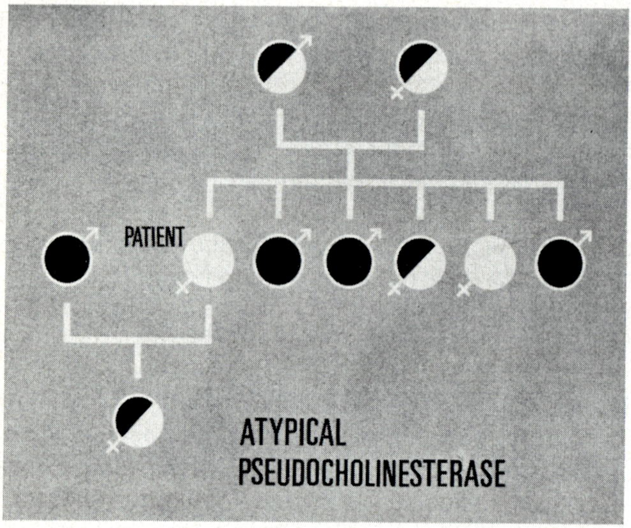

FIG. 129

Family tree demonstrating the genetic linkage of the condition of atypical pseudocholinesterase. One sister of the patient was also homozygous for the condition while other relatives were heterozygous or normal.

normally low pseudocholinesterase level or a normal amount of a different type of pseudocholinesterase which does not hydrolyse suxamethonium.

A typical family tree demonstrating the genetic aspect of this condition is illustrated (Fig. 129). Some patients are heterozygous for the condition and some homozygous.

The anaesthetist is required to assist all too often nowadays in the resuscitation of victims of drug overdosage. The barbiburates are commonly the drugs taken, although phenothiazines, " tranquillisers ", aspirin and occasionally opiates are responsible for the symptoms. In mild cases, the only treatment required, in addition to any specific antidote, is the routine posturing of the patient in the comparatively safe tonsillar position to avoid aspiration of regurgitated stomach contents. A further measure is intubation of the stomach and gastric lavage not only in an attempt to recover any drug which may not yet have been absorbed but also to empty the stomach and again obviate regurgitation of its contents. A word of warning is in order here since it is all too easy, in an unconscious patient, to intubate the lungs and drown the patient during the " gastric " lavage. It is advisable, wherever possible, to carry out endotracheal intubation with a cuffed tube prior to the attempt at lavage. This also enables endotracheal suction to be carried out and guarantees an unobstructed airway during the patient's recovery.

In more severe cases, the clinical state of the patient may warrant other, more active, measures. Severe respiratory depression must be treated by assisted ventilation. This is done in the usual way via a cuffed endotracheal tube delivering oxygen either manually or by a mechanical ventilator. Forced diuresis or dialysis with the artificial kidney may be employed in suitable cases but close attention must always be paid to the patient's respiratory and cardiovascular condition, throughout the period of drug action. Such energetic measures are time-consuming and require the services of skilled nursing and medical personnel and an intensive care unit is the ideal place to treat those severely ill patients.

5. Other Diseases presenting Respiratory Problems

The anaesthetist may be required to assist in the treatment of certain medical conditions where interference with normal respiration is a feature. The disturbance of respiratory function may be a direct result of the disease as in poliomyelitis, polyneuritis or myasthenia gravis, where weakness and paralysis of the respiratory musculature exists, On the other hand, in diseases such as tetanus or status epilepticus, there may be temporary interference with respiration during the convulsions.

Mechanical assistance to ventilation may be required for long periods where there is respiratory paralysis and usually these patients have had a tracheostomy performed. The management of such cases is well understood and can be undertaken in the intensive care unit or the respiratory unit of an infectious diseases hospital. Control of the convulsions of severe tetanus or status epilepticus can be accomplished by administering muscle relaxants and, in this way, the management of the patient becomes similar to that of the paralysed patient with poliomyelitis. A preliminary tracheostomy is usually necessary and the airway is thus safeguarded from danger of obstruction and oxygenation and carbon dioxide elimination assured. This method of treatment avoids the dangers of acute hypoxic incidents which can result in cerebral damage or death in severe tetanus and status epilepticus. Specific therapy for the particular condition must be simultaneously carried out. In the case of tetanus this is the administration of antibiotics and anti-tetanic serum and in the case of status epilepticus treatment with diazepam, sodium phenobarbitone or phenytoin (Epanutin). Controlled ventilation is continued until convulsions cease and thereafter normal spontaneous respiration is permitted.

It can be seen that the anaesthetist can be of assistance to his surgical and medical colleagues in many widely differing circumstances.

CHAPTER XIX

MISHAPS AND THEIR MEDICO-LEGAL ASPECTS

by

ALEX. C. FORRESTER,
M.B., CH.B., F.R.C.S.(G.), F.F.A.R.C.S.

Professor of Anaesthetics, University of Glasgow.
Consultant in Charge, Department of Anaesthetics, Royal Infirmary, Glasgow.

In the practice of anaesthesia, resuscitation, and intensive care, many mishaps may overtake a doctor unless he is constantly on the alert. While a number of these unfortunate occurrences lie within the province of the specialist anaesthetist, some may be encountered by a student or resident, and are included in this chapter to illustrate the hazards which may face them. At the present time, there is an increasing tendency for patients to seek redress at law for any untoward incident which may occur, and it is essential to take adequate precautions when undertaking any procedure known to be associated with complications. A doctor cannot be held to be negligent if he has exercised a reasonable degree of skill and care, no matter what accident has occurred. In the same way, the occurrence of a well recognised hazard does not of itself constitute negligence.

The mishaps to be considered fall conveniently into groups.

Mishaps Associated with Injections

1. INTRA-ARTERIAL THIOPENTONE. Mention has been made in an earlier chapter (p. 91) of the effects of injecting thiopentone into the perivenous tissues or into an artery.

The following case histories illustrate what may happen when an intra-arterial injection of thiopentone is given.

Case 1.—A male patient, aged 38, suffering from hypotension and shock was being anaesthetised. After the usual precautions had been taken, 2 ml. of 5 per cent. thiopentone were injected into a vessel in the medial antecubital fossa. After a pause, during which no pain was experienced, a further 2 ml. were injected. Only then did the patient complain of pain. This was localised to the site of injection and passed off within a minute. Although a small flushed spot developed over the vessel, no other abnormality was noticed and anaesthesia was induced. It was considered that only a slight perivenous leakage had occurred and the surgeon proceeded with the operation. Twenty minutes later, patchy cyanosis was noted in the left forearm and the full picture of an arterial occlusion developed over the next sixteen hours. In spite of all methods of treatment, recognised at the time, including intra-arterial tolazoline and procaine, brachial plexus and stellate ganglion block, heparinisation and arteriotomy, a below elbow amputation was necessary.

This case emphasises the increased risk of accidental intra-arterial injection of thiopentone in shocked patients. With impaired circulation, pulsation will be diminished and the onset of pain may be delayed.

Case 2.—A healthy woman, aged 32, for ligation of varicose veins was given 1·5 ml. of 5 per cent. thiopentone into a vessel in the back of the hand. Agonising, burning pain was experienced in the wrist and hand, accompanied by intense blanching of the ulnar two thirds of the dorsum of the hand and proximal dorsal surfaces of the medial two fingers. Following intra- and peri-arterial procaine, 5 ml. of 1 per cent. by each route, recovery occurred within ten minutes, the intense blanching being followed by reactive hyperaemia.

Although choosing an injection site on the back of the hand does not obviate the risk of intra-arterial injection, tissue necrosis is less likely to occur as there is an extensive collateral circulation in this area. In the unlikely event of an end-artery being entered, at worst only a finger might be lost. By avoiding the medial antecubital fossa, damage to the median nerve is also eliminated.

In addition to avoiding the antecubital fossa one should as a routine ask if the patient feels pain locally or distal to the injection site after injection of 1-2 ml. of solution. In 1962 an anaesthetist was found negligent where he had failed to ask this question and only won his appeal because no pain had been felt.

The routine use of 2·5 per cent. solution of thiopentone is also highly desirable. Experimentally, it has been shown that, using the same total dose of thiopentone intra-arterial injection of 10 per cent. solution, invariably produces gangrene, 5 per cent. almost invariably so while 2·5 per cent. solution never does. Clinically only one case of gangrene has been reported following intra-arterial injection of 2·5 per cent. thiopentone.

At one time the use of 2·5 per cent. solution was decried because the pH of the 5 per cent. and 2·5 per cent. solutions are similar—both over 10, and it was thought that the alkalinity of the solution which caused arterial spasm was responsible for the gangrene which followed.

This has now been disproved and the thiopentone itself is responsible by causing intimal damage and subsequent thrombosis.

Methohexitone 1 per cent. and propanidid 5 per cent. are less irritant even than 2·5 per cent. thiopentone.

The methods of treatment of this accident are summarised in Figure 130.

Treatment of Intra-arterial Thiopentone

1. Postpone operation if possible.
2. Heparinisation.
3. Procaine or tolazoline.
4. Brachial-plexus block.
5. Direct surgical treatment.
   (*a*) Arteriotomy.
   (*b*) Streptokinase infusion.

FIG. 130

Treatment directed solely to the relief of arterial spasm is therefore of limited value. If, however, a very small amount of thiopentone has been given say 0·5-1 ml. of 2·5 per cent. solution, and the accident is recognised immediately, it may be sufficient to inject procaine or tolazoline (Priscol) in and around the artery, with or without sympathetic block, with the object of relieving arterial spasm. If this is successful, as noted by the return of circulation to the part concerned, the anaesthetic and operation may proceed. An inhalational anaesthetic, such as nitrous oxide/oxygen/halothane, may be preferred for induction.

In many cases, however, it will be evident that the circulation is impaired and in these cases in addition to the other measures, it is wise to postpone the operation if at all possible, to allow full heparinisation to be carried out. The usual dose for this is 3 mg./Kg. (300 units/Kg.). This offers the best chance of avoiding necrosis. A special difficulty presents itself when the operation to be performed is an acute emergency when it may be undesirable to postpone operation for more than an hour or two if at all. It has been suggested that in these cases it may be worth giving a smaller dose of heparin, say 1 ml./ Kg. followed, if necessary at the end of the operation by protamine sulphate.

In spite of the above treatment the artery may become thrombosed and the circulation interrupted completely. In the past arteriotomy and removal of the thrombus has been tried with little or no success. More recently the continuous infusion of streptokinase, to digest the fibrin has been successfully used in the treatment of arterial thrombus. This treatment is worthy of consideration in suitable cases.

THE UNCERTAIN RESULTS OF THE TREATMENT OF THIS CONDITION EMPHASISE AGAIN THE EXTREME IMPORTANCE OF PROPHYLAXIS.

2. Indirect Arterial Damage. Apart from damage to an artery by injecting an irritant drug into it, it is possible to cause damage to the artery by injecting a drug close to it.

In one case, hydroxydione was injected into a large vein in the antecubital fossa, and severe spasm of the brachial artery followed, resulting in amputation of the arm. Examination of the limb revealed no direct arterial damage or clotting and the spasm was considered to be due to perivenous leakage of the hydroxydione. In a second patient, injection of hydroxydione into an intravenous infusion at the wrist caused transient spasm of the radial artery.

It is also possible to deposit an irritant solution close to an artery by intramuscular injection, and gangrene of the arm has been reported following intramuscular injection of chlorpromazine in the upper arm close to the brachial artery.

3. Damage to the Median Nerve. In the antecubital fossa the median nerve lies close to the median cubital vein (Fig. 131), and is at risk if an injection is made in this area.

The following case illustrates this danger.

Case 3.—A woman of 40 years was admitted for repair of a hernia. A needle, with a syringe attached, containing 10 ml. of thiopentone 5 per cent. was inserted into an antecubital vein in the left arm and venous blood aspirated. After one ml. was injected the patient complained of some pain at the site of injection and a tingling sensation and numbness of the fingers of the hand. The needle was withdrawn and anaesthesia induced with nitrous oxide and oxygen.

On regaining consciousness the patient experienced loss of sensation in the fingers and palm accompanied by weakness in her hand; a median nerve palsy had resulted. Although she had a repair of the damaged nerve she was left with permanently defective sensation in her thumb and fingers and difficulty in handling objects with her left hand.

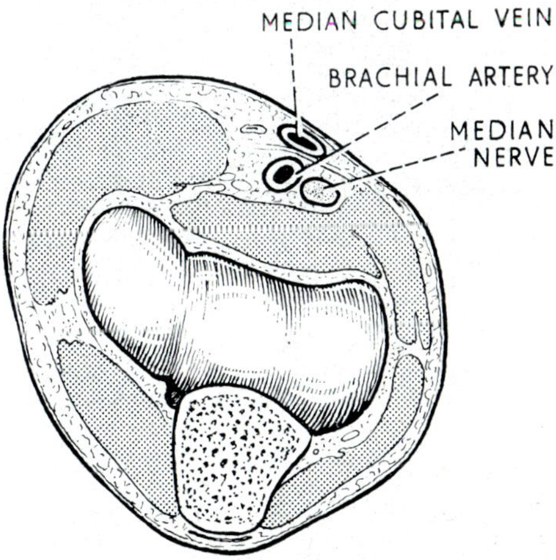

FIG. 131
A section of the antecubital fossa showing the proximity of the brachial artery and median nerve to the median cubital vein.

The close proximity of the median nerve to the antecubital vein was pointed out by Pask and Robson in 1954. They were of the opinion that slight movement of the patient's arm might advance a needle from the vein to the nerve, and it follows that it is wiser to make injections in some other region.

4. LOCAL INJECTION OF VASOCONSTRICTORS. The danger of injecting solutions containing adrenaline in the vicinity of an

end artery has been stressed (p. 228), particularly in the presence of local infection. The oxygen demand of the tissues is increased and when the blood supply is reduced gangrene may result. Figure 132 shows gangrene of a thumb following a ring block using procaine with 1 : 30,000 adrenaline.

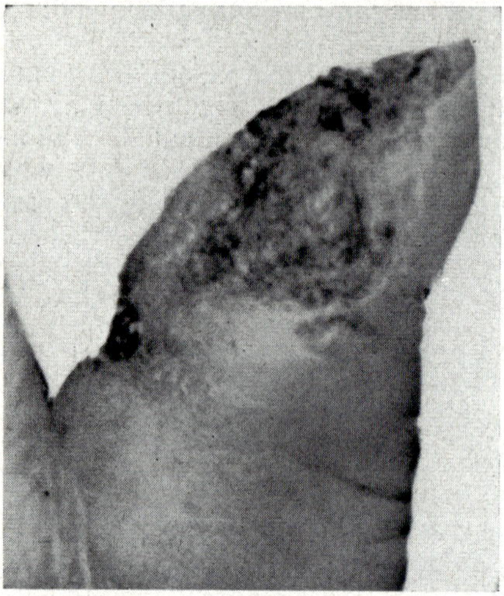

FIG. 132
Gangrene resulting from injection of local analgesic solution containing adrenaline at the base of the thumb.

5. SYSTEMIC USE OF VASOCONSTRICTORS. Noradrenaline infusions are used in patients with severe hypotension arising from different causes. Many of these patients are in a critical condition and often the infusion is made through a drip, set up for other purposes, often in the hand or arm. The danger of using such a peripheral vein for these vasoconstrictors is shown in Figures 133 and 134. Here gangrene of the hand and forearm are shown where these areas have been used. This is caused by the intense local vasoconstriction which is caused by the noradrenaline and, when such a drug is administered, a polythene cannula should be inserted until its tip lies within a large free running vein. This will cause rapid dilution of the drug.

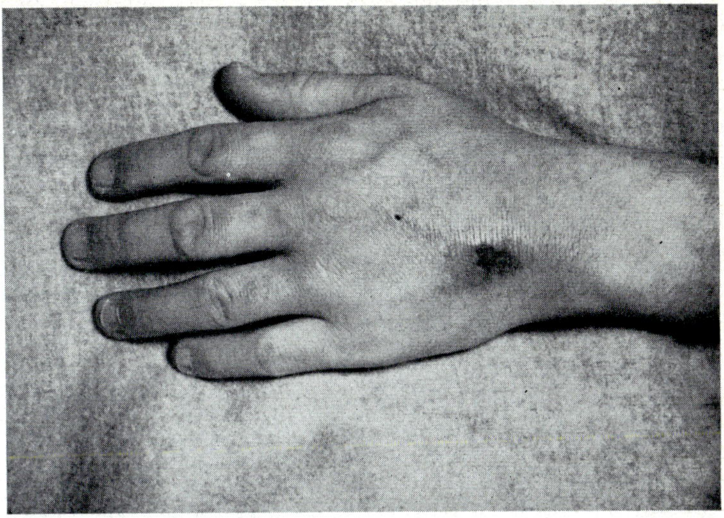

FIG. 133
Skin necrosis following noradrenaline infusion into a vein on the dorsum of the hand.

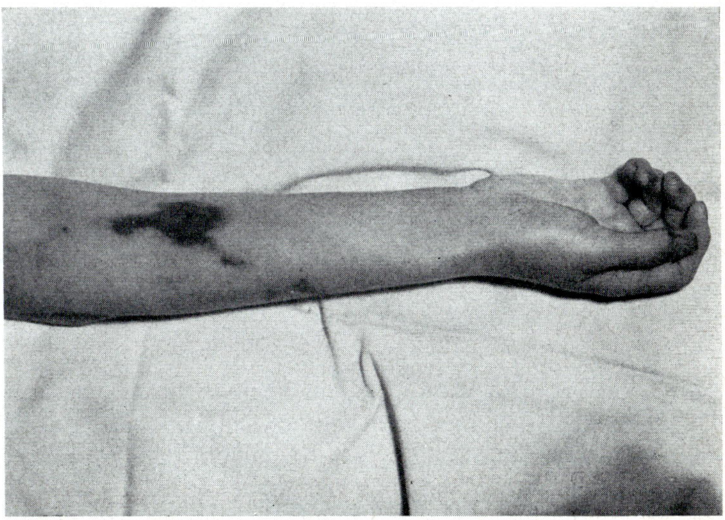

FIG. 134
Skin necrosis following noradrenaline infusion into a vein in the forearm.

If the skin overlying the vein shows colour changes other than slight blanching, the infusion should be stopped at once. Procaine or tolazoline injected into the vein may minimise the vasoconstriction. Nevertheless, two cases have been reported where polythene tubes were inserted fifteen and eight inches respectively into a large vein. Ulcers occurred in both cases at the tips of the cannulae. It may be that these infusions should be administered into the vena cava. Should ischaemia of the skin occur, the use of piperoxamine hydrochloride has been suggested to counteract this, 5 mg. in 20 ml. saline being injected around the vein.

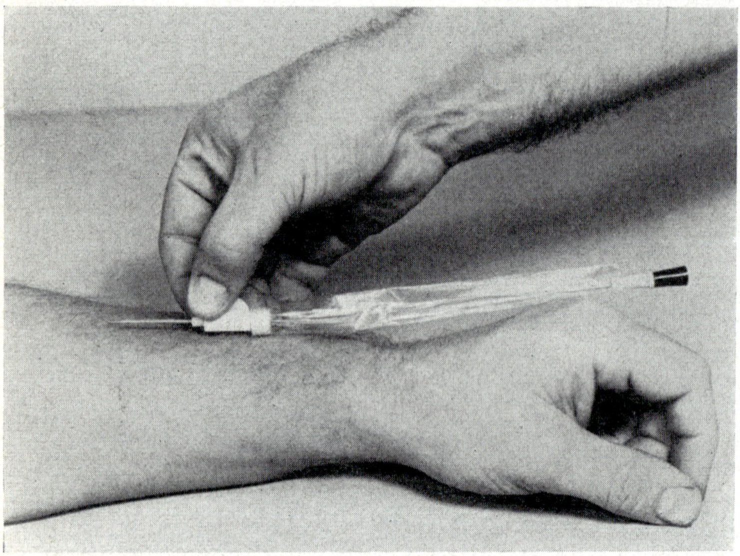

FIG. 135
The Deseret E-Z catheter unit.

6. THE DISAPPEARING CATHETER. The advantage of placing a polythene catheter in a vein without exposing and tying off the vein is considerable. One method of doing this is to insert a metal needle through which a polythene cannula is inserted. This technique has however brought its own hazards and if the polythene catheter is withdrawn through the needle it may be cut on the sharp edge and a portion of catheter left lying

free in the vein. This in turn may migrate towards the heart with serious consequences. This type of set has now been modified. A new approach is that shown in Figure 135 where the needle is inside the plastic catheter and after insertion is withdrawn by means of a stilette.

7. THE WRONG SOLUTION. Great care must be taken to ensure that the solution to be injected, in whatever site, is that which it is intended to use. If the solution comes from a bottle or ampoule, check it with the label or engraving on the ampoule. Do not use fluid from an unlabelled ampoule or bottle either direct or to mix with powder or crystals. This habit has resulted in procaine crystals being mixed with an unlabelled solution which was in fact 1:1,500 cinchocaine. Another accident is illustrated by Case 4.

Case 4.—A brachial plexus block was being performed to remove a piece of metal from the hand. The house surgeon put surgical spirit in one galley pot for cleansing the skin while the anaesthetist prepared lignocaine 2 per cent. in a similar galley pot. Unfortunately, the skin was cleaned with the lignocaine and the spirit was used for injection.

After 9 ml. had been injected the mistake was noticed. The anaesthetist diluted the spirit by injecting into the same area a large quantity of very dilute lignocaine. Analgesia was complete and the foreign body was removed. About two days later, it was apparent that damage had been done to the brachial plexus. The patient was left with considerable disability including stiffness of the joints with muscular weakness and disturbed sensation.

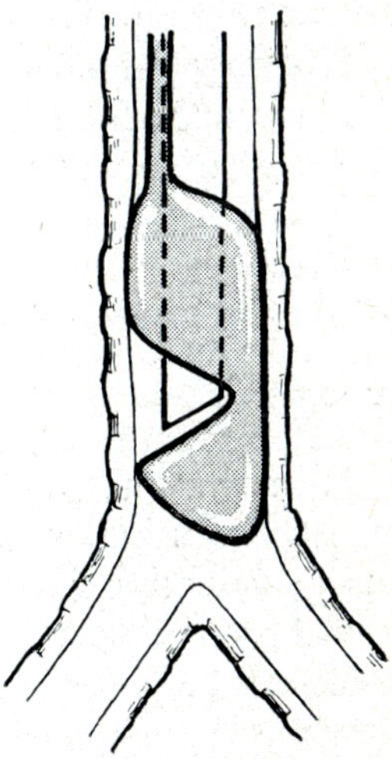

FIG. 136
A diagram illustrating the herniation of the cuff over the end of an endotracheal tube, resulting in respiratory obstruction.

Mishaps due to Respiratory Obstruction

Endotracheal anaesthesia is frequently employed to ensure a free airway. The use of an endotracheal tube does not, however, guarantee that respiratory obstruction will not take place. It has been shown that under certain circumstances tubes may kink, become blocked, or dislodged. A death has occurred following herniation of the cuff over the end of an endotracheal tube (Fig. 136).

Case 5.—A lady of 38 years was undergoing an operation for excision of a cervical rib. A cuffed endotracheal tube was passed and the patient was then turned into the prone position. Spontaneous respiration was satisfactory for half an hour, then movement of the reservoir bag ceased. The cause of the respiratory obstruction was later found to be herniation of the cuff over the end of the tube. This may have been caused by a steady traction on the tube due to the weight of the corrugated tubing and connections. The patient died ten days later from the results of cerebral hypoxia.

Case 6.—A somewhat similar accident occurred when using a latex armoured tube. The herniation developed internally obstructing the lumen completely when the cuff was fully inflated. Fortunately, however, in this case the anaesthetist deflated the cuff and the obstruction was immediately relieved.

The use of disposable plastic endotracheal tubes may be the answer to this problem.

Probably the most common mishap in endotracheal anaesthesia is accidental intubation of the right main bronchus due to the use of too long an endotracheal tube.

Case 7.—Figure 137 shows a tube in the right bronchus with total collapse of the left lung. The bifurcation of the trachea is never lower than the upper border of the 5th thoracic vertebra. The tube here extends to at least the lower border of the 5th vertebra. There is also narrowing of the rib spaces, and mediastinal shift to the collapsed side.

In this case the accident was noticed only at the completion of the operation, when breathing became inadequate. Blood gas examination revealed a Pa_{CO_2} of 100 mm. Hg. Following bronchoscopy, suction and assisted ventilation for about two hours, the patient made a complete recovery.

While the emphasis has here been placed on endotracheal tubes, the resident in an Intensive Care Unit should always be aware of the dangers attendant on the displacement of a tracheostomy tube, or its obstruction by inspissated mucus.

Vomiting during Anaesthesia

Despite the attention which has been focused on the problem, deaths from inhalation of vomitus still occur. A

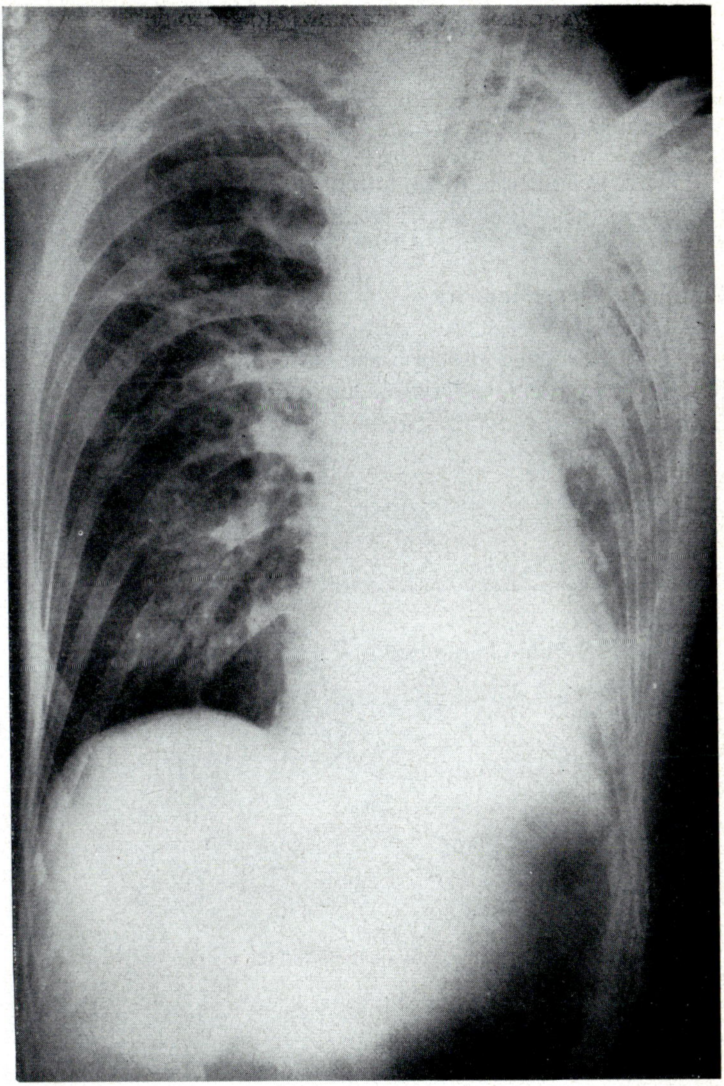

FIG. 137

A radiogram showing an endotracheal tube in the right main bronchus and collapse of the left lung.

recent death resulted from lack of liaison between the anaesthetist, surgeon and nursing staff.

Case 8.—A patient was admitted to hospital for possible Caesarean section. Two hours later she was given a full meal, unknown to the anaesthetist and surgeon. One hour after this, anaesthesia was induced with thiopentone. In the course of induction the patient vomited and, despite all efforts, died shortly afterwards from asphyxia.

This case gave rise to litigation and emphasises the need for full co-operation between nursing and medical staff (Chapter IV).

Peripheral Nerve Injuries

Although spontaneous nerve injuries do occur, damage usually follows the use of unsuitable tourniquets or posture. Recently a patient suffered a median and radial nerve palsy following the use of an Esmarch bandage on the upper arm.

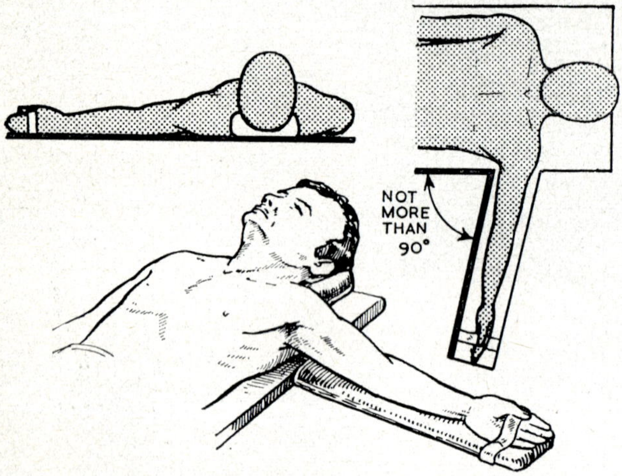

FIG. 138
The correct position of the arm board is shown.

It would appear wise in applying tourniquets to follow the recommendations described below:—

1. In the upper arm, a pneumatic cuff should be routinely employed.
2. In the lower limb, if an Esmarch bandage is used, it should be applied only in the mid-thigh and then only over a towel.

3. The maximum period of application should not be longer than two hours.
4. Precautions should be instituted which will guarantee the removal of the tourniquet at the end of the operation, e.g. tourniquet tied to the table.

The other form of nerve injury associated with operation and anaesthesia is damage to the brachial plexus by incorrect positioning of the arms during infusion (the correct position is shown in Figure 138), or by the incorrect use of shoulder rests. This latter difficulty can be overcome by use of non-slip corrugated mattresses (Fig. 139).

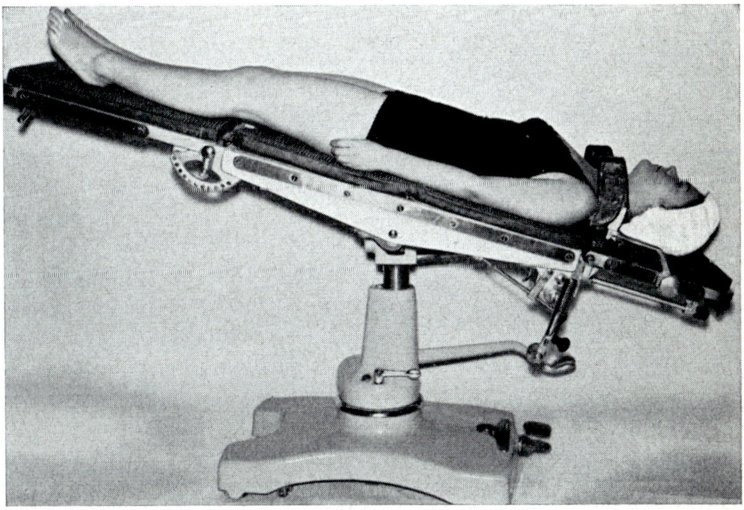

FIG. 139

The Trendelenburg position: the non-slip mattress shown here is of itself sufficient to prevent the patient sliding off the table. The shoulder rests, shown in use here, are essential if a plain mattress is used, but these must be positioned in such a way that damage to the brachial plexus is avoided.

These mishaps are associated with techniques which are in widespread use and are often life saving. Their occurrence should not detract from the techniques, but rather ensure scrupulous care in their application.

Explosions

While explosions in the operating theatre are less common now than when ethers were more widely used the attention of all persons working in the anaesthetic room and operating theatre should be drawn to the potential hazards (see Warning Notice p. 273).

SCOTTISH HOME AND HEALTH DEPARTMENT
FIRES AND EXPLOSIONS IN OPERATING THEATRES AND ANAESTHETIC ROOMS

WARNING NOTICE

Flammable anaesthetic agents such as ether, cyclopropane and ethyl chloride when mixed with air, oxygen or nitrous oxide may form explosive mixtures, and the ignition of such anaesthetic vapours has resulted in explosions which have been attended by serious consequences. The chief causes of such ignitions are : —

(a) Electrostatic spark discharge. This is more likely to occur during dry atmospheric conditions and in particular during the early part of a session when conditions tend to be driest.

(b) Sparking at electrical contacts, diathermy electrodes etc.

(c) Use of apparatus incorporating hot surfaces, e.g. cautery, electric heaters, overheated lamps.

(d) Gas or spirit burners.

Whenever an explosive mixture is in use the surgeon and the theatre sister should be aware of the fact.

PRECAUTIONS AND RECOMMENDATIONS

1. Anti-Static Precautions

The best means of reducing electrostatic risks is to eliminate the use of materials which readily electrify in normal use. *The chief sources of static electricity are insulating rubber, plastics, wool, nylon.* Experience suggests that non-conducting rubber breathing equipment on anaesthetic apparatus constitutes the greatest risk. Materials which are anti-static for practical purposes are available, e.g. anti-static rubber, anti-static rubber-proofed fabrics, linen, cotton and viscose, and should be used wherever possible instead of the electrostatic materials.

Recommended anti-static precautionary measures : —

(a) *Rubberised anaesthetic breathing equipment and rubber tubing* used with suction apparatus, etc., should have permanent anti-static properties.

(b) *Operating tables, anaesthetic apparatus, patients' and other trolleys, stools, etc.*, should have metal or anti-static rubber-tyred castors or feet. The metal work of anaesthetic and other apparatus should be electrically continuous and top surfaces and shelves should be free from paint or other insulating finish.

(c) *Rubber pads* on operating tables, trolleys or stools should have permanent anti-static properties or be completely enclosed in an anti-static fabric, e.g. cotton, linen or viscose rayon.

(d) *All persons entering an anaesthetising location should wear anti-static footwear and a reasonably close-fitting outer garment of an anti-static fabric.* Anti-static rubber-soled footwear is considered preferable. Other types should be enclosed in overboots of an anti-static fabric, e.g. cotton or linen.

(e) Floors should have suitable permanent anti-static properties, e.g. anti-static quality terrazzo, terrazzo tile, P.V.C. or ceramic tile floors.

2. Electrical Apparatus

(a) SWITCH CONTACTS and other parts of apparatus capable of producing an incendive spark should be housed in a gas-tight enclosure or spaced at least four feet horizontally from any anaesthetic apparatus.

(b) The maximum *voltage* of circuits used for energising endoscopes, etc., should be as *low* as is practicable and not appreciably higher than the rated voltage of the lamps. The provision of a special current limiting resistance in the circuit will greatly reduce the spark and overheating risks. *Dry-cell batteries* are safer than mains transformers for operating endoscopes.

(c) *Electrically operated suction apparatus* should have no sparking contacts which are open to atmosphere, and the exhaust outlet from the pump should terminate outside any enclosure housing the apparatus.

(d) From the electrical safety aspect *surgical tools* operated by means of compressed air are considered preferable to electrically-operated tools, because of the inherent spark and electric shock risks associated with the latter.

(e) Flexible *cables* should be free from joints, frequently inspected and renewed when damaged or showing signs of deterioration.

(f) The risks associated with *diathermy and cautery apparatus* are obvious. Before these are used following the administration of flammable anaesthetics a non-flammable gas should be passed through the breathing circuit until no explosive residue remains either in the apparatus or in the patient's lungs. The ether bottle and cyclopropane cylinder should be removed. It is not sufficient to rely on turning these taps off as they might not be gastight.

3. **Open Flames and Heated Surfaces**

Apparatus incorporating open flame burners or heated surfaces which may operate at temperatures of 350°F or more can constitute an ignition risk if located within 20 feet of an anaesthetising position. Doors between the anaesthetising position and the ignition risk should not be regarded as a reliable safeguard, as they may be left open.

NOTES—Spirit lotions, etc. It should be noted that the use of spirit, spirit lotions and other flammable solutions which are frequently employed for cleansing the patient's skin, etc., involves dangers similar to those mentioned above. Additional information on the risks referred to above, together with recommended precautions against associated risks, are contained in "Report of a Working Party on Anaesthetic Explosions" and Hospital Technical Memoranda Nos. 1 and 2 (H.M.S.O.).

Further Safety Precautions

In addition, there must be no smoking in the anaesthetic room or theatre precincts and *all theatre personnel* must be aware when an explosive mixture is in use. In any location where oxygen is being administered the precautions outlined in the warning notice should be observed. This applies equally to areas in general wards.

RECOMMENDED READING

The reader may wish to study certain aspects of anaesthesia in more detail. In this event, the following list of reference books, although by no means exhaustive, may prove helpful.

A Synopsis of Anaesthesia. Lee, J. A., Atkinson, R. S. (1968). 6th edition. John Wright & Sons, Bristol.

Automatic Ventilation of the Lungs. Mushin, W. W., Rendell-Baker, L., Thompson, P. W., Mapelson, W. W. (1969). 2nd edition. Blackwell, Oxford.

Drugs in Anaesthetic Practice. Wood-Smith, F. S., Stewart, H. C., Vickers, M. D. (1968). 3rd edition. Butterworth, London.

Endotracheal Anaesthesia. Gillespie, N. A. (1963). 3rd edition. University of Wisconsin Press, Madison.

General Anaesthesia. Gray, T. C. and Nunn, J. F. (1971). 3rd edition. Butterworth, London.

Introduction to Anaesthesia. Dripps, R. D., Eckenhoff, J. E., Vandam, L. D. (1968). 3rd edition. Saunders, Philadelphia.

Local Anaesthesia: Brachial Plexus. Macintosh, Sir Robert, Mushin, W. W. (1954). 3rd edition. E. & S. Livingstone Ltd., Edinburgh and London.

Lumbar Puncture and Spinal Analgesia. Macintosh, Sir Robert (1957). 2nd edition. E. & S. Livingstone Ltd., Edinburgh and London.

Oxford Handbooks for Medical Auxiliaries: Anaesthetics. Vaughan A. B. (1969). Oxford University Press.

Paediatric Anaesthesia. Davenport, H. T. (1967). Heinemann, London.

Principles and Practice of Obstetric Anaesthesia. Crawford, J. S. (1965). 2nd edition. Blackwell Scientific Publications, Oxford.

Respiratory Failure. Campbell, E. J. M., Sykes, M. K., McNicol, M. W. (1969). Blackwell, London.

Spinal Epidural Analgesia. Bromage, P. R. (1954). E. & S. Livingstone Ltd., Edinburgh and London.

The Lung. Comroe, J. H., Forster, R. E., Dubois, A. B., Briscoe, W. A., Carlsen, E. (1967). 2nd edition. Year Book Medical Publishers Inc., Chicago.

INDEX

The Central Press (Aberdeen) Ltd., Belmont St., Aberdeen.